CARDIAC REHABILITATION

CLINICS IN PHYSICAL THERAPY
VOLUME 1

Forthcoming Volumes in the Series

Vol. 2 Electrotherapy
Steven L. Wolf, Ph.D., guest editor

Vol. 3 Physical Therapy Practice in Community Health Settings
Jane S. Mathews, Ph.D., guest editor

Vol. 4 Mobilization of the Shoulder
Sandy Burkart, Ph.D., guest editor

Vol. 5 Neurological Pathokinesiology in the Adult
Shirley Sahrmann, Ph.D., guest editor

Vol. 6 Physical Therapy of the Geriatric Patient
Osa Littrup Jackson, Ph.D., guest editor

Vol. 7 Rehabilitation of the Burn Patient
Vincent DiGregorio, M.D., guest editor

CARDIAC REHABILITATION

Edited by

Louis R. Amundsen, R.P.T., Ph.D.

Director of Graduate Study
Course in Physical Therapy
Department of Physical Medicine and Rehabilitation
University of Minnesota
Minneapolis, Minnesota

CHURCHILL LIVINGSTONE
NEW YORK, EDINBURGH, LONDON AND MELBOURNE
1981

© Churchill Livingstone Inc. 1981

Distributed in the United Kingdom by Churchill Livingstone, Robert Stevenson House, 1–3 Baxter's Place, Leith Walk, Edinburgh EH1 3AF and by associated companies, branches and representatives throughout the world.

First published 1981

Printed in USA

ISBN 0–443–08147–6

7 6 5 4 3 2 1

Library of Congress Cataloging in Publication Data
Main entry under title:

Cardiac rehabilitation.

    (Clinics in physical therapy; v. 1)
    Bibliography: p.
    Includes index.
    Contents: Normal and abnormal cardio-
vascular responses to acute physical exercise /
Louis R. Amundsen and David H. Nielsen—
Exercise physiology / David H. Nielsen and
Louis R. Amundsen—Physiological effects of
endurance training / Terry Hoskins Michel—
[etc.]
    1. Exercise therapy. 2. Cardiacs—Rehabil-
itation. I. Amundsen, Louis R. II. Series.
RC684.E9C37   616.1'2062   81-10270
ISBN 0-443-08147-6   AACR2

Contributors

Louis R. Amundsen, R.P.T., Ph.D.
Director of Graduate Study, Course in Physical Therapy, Department of Physical Medicine and Rehabilitation, University of Minnesota, Minneapolis, Minnesota

Lois M. Canafax, R.P.T., B.S.
Physical Therapy Supervisor, Methodist Hospital, St. Louis Park, Minnesota

Charles L. Carter, L.P.T., Ph.D.
Assistant Professor, School of Physical Therapy, University of Southern California, Downey, California

Kathleen Marie Janikula Fleischaker, R.P.T., B.S.
Clinical Faculty, Course in Physical Therapy, University of Minnesota Medical School; Clinical Instructor, P.T.A. Program, St. Mary's Junior College; Clinical Instructor, College of St. Scholastica; Director of Rehabilitation Services, Methodist Hospital, St. Louis Park, Minnesota

Mary A. Gower, R.P.T., B.S.
Registered Physical Therapist, Methodist Hospital, St. Louis Park, Minnesota

Robin S. Graf, R.P.T., M.S.
Clinical Faculty, University of Southern California; Lecturer, Children's Hospital School of Physical Therapy; Program Director, Cardiac Rehabilitation, California Primary Physicians; Cardiopulmonary Clinical Specialist, California Hospital Medical Center, Los Angeles, California

Louise June Holt, R.N., B.S.
Cardiac Outpatient Registered Nurse, Methodist Hospital, St. Louis Park, Minnesota

Stuart L. Lowenthal, L.P.T., B.S.
Director, Diagnostic Exercise Laboratory and Cardiac Rehabilitation Program, Heart, Inc., Lexington, Kentucky

Brenda Rae Lunsford, M.S., R.P.T.
Physical Therapy Supervisor II, Rancho Los Amigos Hospital, Downey, California

R. G. McAllister, Jr., M.D., F.A.C.C.
Associate Professor of Medicine, (Cardiology) and Pharmacology, University of Kentucky College of Medicine; Associate Chief of Staff/Research, Veterans Administration Medical Center, Lexington, Kentucky

Theresa Hoskins Michel, R.P.T., M.S.
Research Associate, Department of Physical Medicine and Rehabilitation, Tufts New England Medical Center, Boston, Massachusetts

David H. Nielsen, L.P.T., Ph.D.
Associate Professor, Physical Therapy Education, University of Iowa, Iowa City, Iowa

Marcia J. Pearl, M.A., R.P.T.
Senior Associate, Division of Physical Therapy, Department of Community Health, Emory University School of Medicine; Consultant, Physical Therapy Department, Crawford Long Hospital, Atlanta, Georgia

Bill Schoneberger, M.S., R.P.T.
Clinical Faculty, School of Physical Therapy, University of Southern California; Physical Therapy Instructor, Rancho Los Amigos Hospital, Downey, California

Marion B. Schoneberger, R.P.T. B.S.
Physical Therapy Supervisor I, Rancho Los Amigos Hospital, Downey, California

Foreword to the Series

The guiding principle of this series, as initially stated by the publisher, is that *Clinics in Physical Therapy* should be written for the practicing physical therapist for the purpose of providing an up-date on current information and an overview of the state of the art in each of several topics in clinical physical therapy. Some volumes will focus on methods of treatment, such as Electrotherapy, while most volumes will relate to particular areas of practice, such as Cardiac Rehabilitation, Geriatric Physical Therapy, or Neurological Problems in Adults.

It is expected that students in professional physical therapy curricula will also find the information in this series useful as they prepare for clinical education and clinical roles as practitioners of physical therapy. Nevertheless, the series is written primarily for clinicians and is meant to provide information useful in daily practice. The publishers and editors hope that readers will provide constructive critiques about the extent to which this purpose is met. Helpful suggestions are welcome, particularly concerning how to improve individual volumes and about areas of practice for which a one-volume source of information is needed.

To be successful, any venture such as *Clinics in Physical Therapy* requires the effort, cooperation, and coordination of a number of people. First, I would like to thank Lewis Reines, President of Churchill Livingstone Inc., who recognized that physical therapy had reached a level of sophistication (that is, knowledge and skills) where it could produce and use a series such as this. His foresight and faith in us is greatly appreciated.

Next, I acknowledge the members of the Editorial Board of *Clinics in Physical Therapy,* Drs. Louis R. Amundsen, Sandy Burkart, Steven L. Wolf, and Shirley Sahrmann. They were chosen for their demonstrated clinical expertise, academic knowledge, and writing and/or editing abilities. With me, they shared responsibility for selecting topics and guest editors for each volume and for approving the table of contents and contributors for each volume. Finally, and most importantly, I would like to acknowledge and thank William R. Schmitt, Senior Medical Editor and Manager of Serial Publications of Churchill Livingstone Inc., whose encouragement, management skills, and attention to detail have made *Clinics in Physical Therapy* a practical reality.

Otto D. Payton, Ph.D.
Chairman, Editorial Advisory Board
Clinics in Physical Therapy

Preface

The need for a single source that would cover the state-of-the-art cardiac rehabilitation has been apparent to me whenever I have assigned or recommended readings for undergraduates, advanced degree students, or continuing education participants. This book is designed to provide that single source of applied science and clinical information.

The content is intended to be relatively comprehensive but not controversial. We have documented our summaries and recommendations, but have not attempted to provide a forum for original research.

The book is organized and written at a level which should be optimal for both the undergraduate student and the practicing clinician. General background information is presented in the first three chapters. This applied science should be relatively easy for physical therapists and other related health professionals to assimilate, and also will have direct and immediate clinical applicability in many instances. A thorough understanding of this material will make the physical therapist a more flexible clinician.

The next three chapters deal with clinical assessment. This coverage is intended to be relatively comprehensive. All physical therapists should not necessarily expect to perform all of the assessments that have been described. For example, in some settings a physical therapist would not be expected to perform or interpret the graded exercise tolerance test. Yet an understanding of this test and the meaning of the results is an integral part of the daily assessment of exercise tolerance and of treatment planning.

The last three chapters cover patient treatment. To provide general and specific guidelines, the general principle of program planning and a specific program example are included. Ideally, the reader of this book will assimilate all parts of the book, his or her unique working situation, and current research reports before writing guidelines for a local program.

Even though my long range goals included writing a book on this topic, it would not have been done at this time without Dr. Otto Payton's request to include this volume in the series *Clinics in Physical Therapy*. The Cardiopulmonary Section of the American Physical Therapy Association made the selection of topics and contributors relatively simple. Authors or coauthors of all chapters are members of this section, and my initial contacts with most of them came about while I attended Cardiopulmonary Section functions. It is my hope that this book will further the goals of this Cardiopulmonary Section, and that it will become a valued resource for anyone involved in cardiac rehabilitation.

Louis R. Amundsen

Contents

CARDIAC REHABILITATION

1 | Normal and Abnormal Cardiovascular Responses to Acute Physical Exercise

Louis R. Amundsen
David H. Nielsen

The cardiovascular and pulmonary systems respond to acute exercise by increasing heart rate, respiratory rate, stroke volume, tidal volume, and blood flow to active tissue. These changes are designed to allow the individual to meet the demands for oxygen and energy substrate as quickly and completely as possible. When work loads are appropriate the physiological systems rapidly reach an equilibrium or steady state condition.[1] During steady state, oxygen and energy substrate delivery equal utilization, and the functional reserve capacities of the cardiovascular and pulmonary systems are not exceeded. At steady state, aerobic metabolism predominates, and exercise can safely be continued for relatively long periods of time. When work loads are continuously increased, each individual will eventually exceed his capacity to achieve a steady state, and will soon be unable to continue to exercise. It is our responsibility to recognize, predict, or prevent exercise or activity intolerance. Even though the dangers of physical exercise are often exaggerated, it is our goal to minimize these dangers and to utilize the most effective levels of exercise for a given patient.

1

RESTING STATE

Prior to initiating any form of exercise the patient must be able to reach steady state conditions at rest. The pulse rate should be between 60 and 100 beats per minute (bpm) and it should be strong and regular. If the rate is outside this range or irregular, cardiac arrhythmias are likely and the electrocardiogram must be obtained or referred to in the medical chart (see Ch. 5 for a discussion of ECG interpretation). The systolic blood pressure should be between 100 and 150 mmHg.[2, 3] Lower pressures are indicative of cardiovascular collapse and higher pressures of hypertension. The respiratory rate should be approximately 12/min, regular, and not labored. The tidal volume should be around 500 ml. The patient should be comfortable and alert. He should have normal facial color: this rules out cyanosis, extreme pallor, or pronounced flushing. Perspiration should be absent unless the ambient temperature is high. A detailed description of what to look for in medical records and how to perform the physical assessment prior to exercise follows in Chapter 4.

CARDIOPULMONARY RESPONSES TO ACUTE PHYSICAL EXERCISE

Normal and abnormal cardiopulmonary responses to exercise can be identified. The primary physiological changes which occur are increases in heart rate, stroke volume, respiratory rate, tidal volume, blood flow to active tissue, and metabolic rate of active tissue.

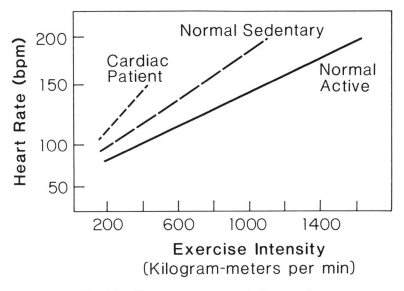

Fig. 1-1.   Heart rate responses during exercise.

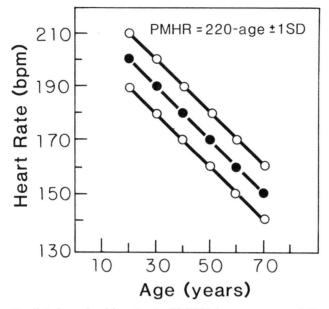

Fig. 1-2. Predicted maximal heart rate (PMHR) in an average adult population.

Heart Rate

The heart rate normally increases as the work rate increases (Fig. 1-1).[4,5] While this increase in heart rate is usually linear, it will be different for each individual. Usually healthier and more active individuals have slower heart rates at any given work rate (Fig. 1-1). However, cardiac patients will have lower maximal heart rates than normal subjects of the same age, and may even have lower heart rates than normal subjects at very low workloads. The predicted maximal heart rate will progressively decrease with increases in age of an average apparently healthy population (Fig. 1-2).[6,7] Occasionally, even in a patient with a normal cardiovascular system, the heart rate will be abnormally high at rest and during low intensity exercise but will be appropriate at higher work rates (Fig. 1-3).[8,9] This response is possible during any diagnostic test, during initial treatment sessions, and whenever audiences suddenly appear or enlarge beyond levels customary for the patient.

One can be most certain of the ability of the patient to reach and maintain steady state conditions at intensities of exercise which cause heart rates to increase to a maximum of 60 to 75 percent of the available heart rate range.[1,7] This recommended training heart rate range can be predicted from estimated resting and maximal heart rates (Fig. 1-4).[7] These training heart rate ranges represent an estimate of the safest effective training intensity. The results of a progressive exercise tolerance test need to be available, however, before training intensities can be established for patients with known cardiac disease (see Chs. 6 and 8).

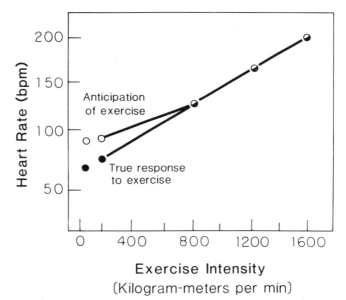

Fig. 1-3. Anticipatory response to exercise versus a purely physiological response to exercise in the same individual.

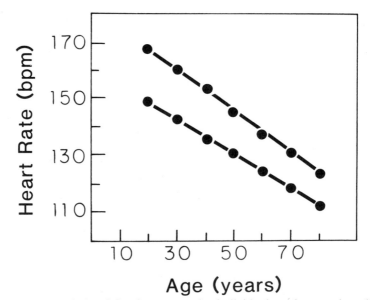

Fig. 1-4. Recommended training heart rates for individuals with normal cardiopulmonary systems. Calculated using Karvonen's formula and a resting heart rate of 70 bpm.

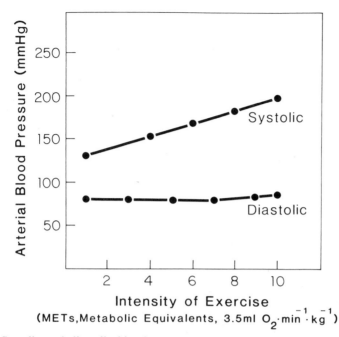

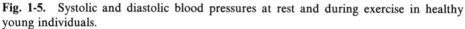

Fig. 1-5. Systolic and diastolic blood pressures at rest and during exercise in healthy young individuals.

Blood Pressure Responses

Blood pressure normally increases linearly as the intensity of exercise increases (Fig. 1-5).[10] Naughton has determined that the normal increase in systolic blood pressure (SBP) is 7.5 mmHg per MET. An increase of less than 5 mmHg per MET is considered a hypotensive response and an increase of greater than 12 mmHg per MET is considered a hypertensive response.[11] When SBP fails to increase as the work load is increased the functional reserve capacity of the heart has usually been exceeded. Exercise intensity should be immediately reduced when SBP falls or fails to increase as the intensity of exercise increases. If the SBP exceeds 225 to 230 mmHg the exercise intensity should be reduced to minimize chances for excessive work of the heart and to reduce the risk of arterial rupture or aneurysm formation.[7]

The diastolic blood pressure normally changes very little during such rhythmic lower extremity exercise as ambulation, bicycling, or treadmill walking. An increase of 20 mmHg has been considered a sign that a patient has exceeded his cardiac reserve capacity and that blood flow to the liver, kidney, and digestive tract is being critically curtailed.[7]

During arm exercise or isometric exercise of any muscle group the systolic and diastolic arterial pressures normally increase.[12, 13] Exercise should be stopped or decreased in intensity if the diastolic pressure exceeds 130 mmHg.[7]

Stroke Volume

During upright exercise, stroke volume should increase from 60 to 80 ml at rest, to 100 to 140 ml at 50 percent of maximal aerobic working capacity, and to 115 to 150 ml at 100 percent of maximal capacity of untrained and highly fit young men, respectively.[6, 9] Cardiac problems, especially ischemic heart disease, will lower resting stroke volumes and will also lower the potential (relatively small even in normal subjects) increase in stroke volume observed during exercise.[4] Data concerning stroke volumes may be available in the medical chart (see Ch. 4). Or, the physical therapist can estimate the relative stroke volume and changes in stroke volume during exercise by observing the pulse pressure (SBP—DBP).[14]

Regional Blood Flow

The tremendous increase in the metabolic rate of skeletal muscle (100×) requires that the percent of total cardiac output, which increases only 12 times, flowing through active skeletal muscle be increased to meet the requirements for oxygen and metabolic substrates (glucose and free fatty acids).[9, 15] The relative changes in absolute blood flow are illustrated in Figure 1-6.[4, 6, 9]

By observing certain signs and symptoms, the clinical physical therapist can estimate the adequacy of regional blood flow. Blood flow to the skin should be sufficient to produce pink cheeks. If the cheeks, nose, and earlobes get progressively pinker as the exercise intensity increases, but suddenly turn pale, the intensity of exercise must be reduced or stopped, especially if the systolic blood pressure is falling and the diastolic pressure is simultaneously increasing. These

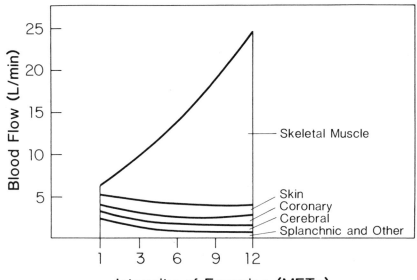

Fig. 1-6.   Regional blood flow during exercise in healthy young adults.

changes indicate that the absolute and relative blood flow to the kidney and liver is being sacrificed to allow blood flow to more critical areas (working muscle, the heart, and the brain).[7] Cognition, coordination, and equilibrium will deteriorate if cerebral blood flow is inadequate. Angina pectoris and ST segment depression on the electrocardiogram will occur if coronary blood flow is inadequate. Inadequate blood flow to active lower extremity skeletal muscles causes claudication.

Pulmonary Ventilation

Minute ventilation should increase as the intensity of exercise increases.[1, 6] The rate of increase in ventilation is greater per unit increase in intensity of exercise for sedentary individuals or for individuals with cardiac disease than it is for healthy trained individuals. This response (Fig. 1-7) is essentially linear at lower intensities of exercise up to 60 to 75 percent of maximal capacity, and non-linear at higher intensities.[6, 16] It becomes more and more difficult to achieve a steady state at the higher exercise intensities. The region where this response becomes curvilinear has been called the anaerobic threshold.[16] This breakpoint occurs at higher points on the line in trained than in untrained individuals. While this relationship is rarely documented clinically, the necessary measurements could be performed with inexpensive equipment. MET levels are almost always available during standardized exercise for cardiac patients, and minute ventilation can be measured with minimal difficulty or expense.

Some of the main stimuli for increasing minute ventilation are believed to be metabolites in active skeletal muscle.[16] When these metabolites begin to accumulate because of a failure of the cardiovascular system, minute ventilation will be

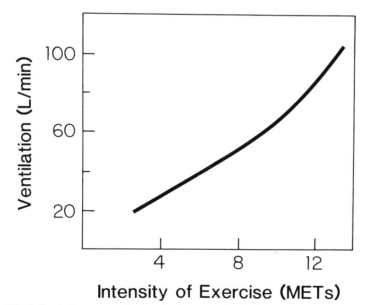

Fig. 1-7. Minute ventilation during exercise in healthy young adults.

increased to uncomfortable levels and dyspnea or shortness of breath will be perceived by the patient.[17]

Arteriovenous Oxygen Content Difference

In normal healthy individuals the arterial oxygen content is optimal ($\sim$20 ml O_2/100 ml blood) and doesn't change as the intensity of exercise increases.[1] Normally the venous oxygen content ($\sim$15 ml O_2/100 ml blood) at rest progressively decreases to as low as 3.5 ml O_2/100 ml blood during maximal exercise. Postmyocardial infarction patients are likely to have normal arteriovenous oxygen content differences, unless they develop congestive heart failure. Sedentary individuals will usually have higher venous oxygen concentrations (less arteriovenous oxygen content difference) during maximal exercise than trained individuals. Patients with vasoregulatory asthenia have less arteriovenous oxygen difference during maximal exercise than normal subjects, because of a failure to optimally increase the proportion of cardiac output flowing through active skeletal muscle.[16]

RECOVERY

The rate of return toward resting levels of the heart rate, blood pressure, and minute ventilation is proportionate to the extent that steady state could be achieved during exercise and conversely to the degree that anaerobic metabolism was utilized during the activity. It has been suggested that the heart rate should be below 110 to 100 bpm 6 minutes after exercise ceases.[18] If dyspnea or angina occurred during exercise, they should rapidly disappear after exercise. Blood pressure should also return rapidly to resting levels; however, precipitous drops in pressure are possible after exercise because of vasodilatation and pooling of blood in the lower extremities.[19] Patients should exercise at low levels during a cool down phase prior to the end of an exercise session. This will help to prevent excessively rapid decreases in blood pressure. Sitting with the feet up is recommended if low-level exercise is not feasible. This position facilitates optimal venous return. The recumbent position is not recommended because venous return may be excessive. Excessive filling of the heart will increase myocardial oxygen cost unnecessarily and can precipitate failure.

CONCLUSIONS

Normally, sufficient cardiopulmonary and metabolic reserves exist to safely permit any intensity of exercise; however, cardiovascular disorders can eliminate all reserve capacity and cause higher intensity activity to be dangerous. The application of the principles outlined in this chapter and in the remainder of this book will help to ensure that exercise can be applied at therapeutic levels to patients with cardiovascular disease.

REFERENCES

1. Åstrand P-O, Rodahl K: Textbook of Work Physiology, New York, McGraw-Hill, 1977
2. Milnor WR: Principles of hemodynamics. In: Medical Physiology, ed. Mountcastle VB. St. Louis, The CV Mosby Company, 1968
3. Bates B: Pressures and pulses: arterial and venous. In: A Guide to Physical Examination. Philadelphia, JB Lippincott, 1979
4. Rowell LB: Human cardiovascular responses to exercise. In: Exercise and the Heart: Guidelines for Exercise Programs, ed. Morse RL. Springfield, IL, Charles C Thomas, 1972
5. Denolin H, Messin R, Degré S: Testing of the working capacity of cardiac patients. In: Physical Activity and the Heart, ed. Karvonen MJ and Barry AJ. Springfield, IL, Charles C Thomas, 1967
6. Jones NL, Campbell EJM, Edwards RHT, et al: Physiology of exercise. In: Clinical Exercise Testing. Philadelphia, WB Saunders, 1975
7. Amundsen LR: Assessing exercise tolerance: a review. Phys Ther 59:534–537, 1979
8. Bruce RA: Principles of exercise testing. In: Exercise Testing and Exercise Training in Coronary Heart Disease, ed. Naughton J and Hellerstein HK. New York, Academic Press, 1973
9. Andersen KL, Shepard RJ, Denolin H, et al: Fundamentals of exercise physiology. In: Fundamentals of Exercise Testing. Geneva, World Health Organization, 1971
10. Carlsten A, Grimby G: Effects of exercise on the central circulation. In: The Circulatory Response to Muscular Exercise in Man. Springfield, IL, Charles C. Thomas, 1966
11. Naughton J, Haider R: Methods of exercise testing. In: Exercise Testing and Exercise Training in Coronary Heart Disease, ed. Naughton J and Hellerstein HK. New York, Academic Press, 1973
12. Åstrand P-O, Ekblom B, Messin R, et al: Intra-arterial blood pressure during exercise with different muscle groups. J Appl Physiol 20:253–256, 1965
13. Donald KW, Lind AR, McNicol GW: Cardiovascular responses to sustained contractions. Cir Res, Suppl 20 and 21:1–15, 1–30, 1967
14. Rushmer RF: The cardiac output. In: Cardiovascular Dynamics. Philadelphia, WB Saunders, 1970
15. Buskirk ER: Cardiovascular adaptation to physical effort in healthy men. In: Exercise Testing and Exercise Training in Coronary Heart Disease, ed. Naughton J and Hellerstein HK. New York, Academic Press, 1973
16. Dempsey JA, Rankin J: Physiologic adaptations of gas transport systems to muscular work in health and disease. Am J Phys Med 46:582–647, 1967
17. Rankin J, Dempsey JA: Respiratory muscles and the mechanisms of breathing. Am J Phys Med 46:198–244, 1967
18. Haskell WL: Design and implementation of cardiac conditioning programs. In: Rehabilitation of the Coronary Patient. New York, John Wiley and Sons, 1978
19. Hellerstein HK, Franklin BA: Exercise testing and prescription. In: Rehabilitation of the Coronary Patient. New York, John Wiley and Sons, 1978

2 Exercise Physiology: An Overview with Emphasis on Aerobic Capacity and Energy Cost

David H. Nielsen
Louis R. Amundsen

Physical inactivity, a cultural by-product of our mechanized society, is often implicated as a possible risk factor of coronary heart disease.[1] Minimizing this risk factor is a primary goal of prevention and rehabilitation programs, even though complete proof of the prophylactic effects of exercise is still lacking.[2] The feasibility and the educational and physiological benefits of physical conditioning for patients with coronary heart disease have been established.[3-9]

The success of rehabilitation programs largely depends upon the ability of the therapist to apply scientifically based rationale to patient evaluation and treatment. A basic understanding of exercise physiology is a necessary prerequisite.

The purpose of this chapter is to provide an overview of background information concerning exercise physiology, including: force, work, and power; energy metabolism; work efficiency; assessment of aerobic capacity; and the energy cost of selected physical activities as they relate to exercise training programs and patient consultation.

FORCE, WORK, AND POWER

In exercising man, force is generated and work is done through muscle contraction and shortening. By definition work is the product of unit force times unit distance ($W = f \cdot d$). The adopted metric unit of work is the kilopond $\cdot$ meter (kpm). Since 1 kp is the force acting on the mass of 1 kilogram (kg) at the normal acceleration of gravity, by convention the units kp and kg and kpm and kgm are used interchangeably. Work load or work rate reflects the work performed per unit time, usually expressed in terms of minutes (min), and can be represented as a power function ($\dot{W} = f \cdot d/t$). The corresponding units are kpm/min and kgm/min. Power is frequently also expressed in electrical units—watts (1 watt = 6.12 kpm/min)—and thermal units—kilocalories per minute (1 kcal/min = 427 kpm/min). In SI Units (Le Système International d'Unités) 1 watt equals 1 joule per sec or 1 newton meter per sec.

ENERGY METABOLISM

There are two general metabolic pathways in the muscle for providing energy for doing work. The distinguishing factor is that one pathway does not require oxygen (anaerobic metabolism) while the other one does (aerobic metabolism). The principal reactions are outlined in Table 2-1.[10-12]

Adenosine triphosphate (ATP) is the intermediary energy compound in the transduction of ingested food energy into the mechanical energy of muscle contraction and work.[11] The energy released in the hydrolysis of the terminal high energy phosphate bond in this compound is utilized in the conformational changes and generation of cross-bridges in the actin and myocin myofilaments which result in tension development and muscle shortening. Resting intramuscular concentrations of ATP are sufficient to meet the energy requirements of the exercising muscle for only a few seconds. The concentration of intramuscular ATP, however, decreases only slightly during exercise because of the continued

Table 2-1. Principal metabolic pathways[10-12]

A. Anaerobic Metabolism (without oxygen)
   1. ATP $\rightleftharpoons$ ADP + P + energy
   2. creatine phosphate + ADP $\rightleftharpoons$ creatine + ATP
   3. glucose or muscle glycogen + P + ADP $\rightarrow$ lactate + ATP[a]
B. Aerobic Metabolism (with oxygen)
   1. glucose or muscle glycogen + P + ADP + O_2 $\rightarrow$ CO_2 + H_2O + ATP[b]
   2. free fatty acids + P + ADP + O_2 $\rightarrow$ CO_2 + H_2O + ATP[c]

[a] Energy yield = 2 ATP/mole of glucose
[b] Energy yield = 38 ATP/mole of glucose
  Oxidative efficiency: 1 mole O_2 $\rightarrow$ 6.5 ATP
[c] Energy yield = 130 ATP/mole FFA (palmitate)
  Oxidative efficiency: 1 mole O_2 $\rightarrow$ 5.7 ATP

regeneration of ATP through transphosphorylation of creatine phosphate (CP).[12] Consequently, intramuscular CP concentration decreases progressively with increases in work rate. The total amount of intramuscular CP is also small. The combined stores of ATP and CP are depleted within less than 10 seconds of maximum intensity exercise.[12] Continued muscular activity requires replenishment of ATP, ultimately through the catabolism of ingested food.

Although each of the three primary food categories, carbohydrates, fat and protein, is capable of being utilized to generate ATP during exercise, protein is generally regarded as an unimportant contributor to skeletal muscle energy metabolism except under conditions of starvation. Glucose, glycogen, and free fatty acids are the major fuels. The selection of fuel and pathway depends upon the duration and intensity of the exercise. Glucose and glycogen may be metabolized either anaerobically or aerobically, while free fatty acid metabolism is strictly oxidative.

As indicated in Table 2-1, the energy yield differs significantly between anaerobic and aerobic metabolism of glucose (2 ATP/mole of glucose versus 38 ATP/mole of glucose) as well as between substrates (38 ATP/mole of glucose versus 130 ATP/mole palmitate).[10-12] The physiological cost of using these substrates differs in the opposite direction. With complete oxidation, palmitate is approximately 88 percent as efficient as glucose in providing energy for work per liter of oxygen consumed. From an energy yield per unit weight point of view, fatty acids are the preferred substrate. Under conditions in which the rate of oxygen uptake may limit the person's ability to perform a physical activity, however, the oxidation of carbohydrate is more beneficial than fatty acid for maximizing energy yield per liter of oxygen consumed.

Through gas exchange measurements and the determination of the respiratory quotient ($RQ = CO_2$ produced$/O_2$ consumed), patterns of substrate utilization during exercise have been studied.[12, 13] The results indicate that free fatty acids are important energy sources during rest and low-level steady state exercise. The proportion of energy derived from carbohydrate increases gradually with increase in intensity of low-level exercise but steeply at effort levels of 65 to 75 percent of the maximal work capacity, as metabolism becomes progressively more anaerobic.[14] Concomitant progressive increases in blood lactate occur above this anaerobic threshold.[15] Only carbohydrates are metabolized during maximal exercise, and at this intensity anaerobic glycolysis provides only enough ATP to sustain the activity for approximately 1 minute before the buildup of lactic acid prohibits further exercise.[12]

WORK EFFICIENCY

Efficiency of the human body relates to the effective function of the cardiopulmonary and musculoskeletal systems in performing specific physical tasks. In physics, mechanical efficiency is defined as the ratio of work output to the work input. The exercise physiologist, however, defines work efficiency (Ew) as the ratio of the work rate to the energy cost (oxygen uptake, $\dot{V}O_2$). Obviously, work rate and energy cost must be expressed in the same units—watts, kpm/min, or kcal/min. The interconversion of mechanical work units was previously considered (1 watt = 6 kpm/min or 1 kpm/min = .17 watts; 1 kpm/min = .00234 kcal/min or 1 kcal/min = 427 kpm/min at 100 percent efficiency). The relative caloric equivalents of fat oxidation (4.70 kcal/liter O_2) and carbohydrate oxidation (5.05 kcal/1 O_2) were also previously discussed. Since carbohydrate is the preferred substrate for exercise, the latter value is conventionally used for estimating the caloric equivalent energy cost of physical activity. The following example illustrates the necessary conversions for the determinations of Ew for exercising on the bicycle ergometer:

$$Ew = \frac{\text{Work rate}}{\text{Energy Cost } (\dot{V}O_2)} = \frac{(kpm/min)\ (.00234\ kcal/kpm)}{(1\ O_2/min)\ (5.05\ kcal/1\ O_2)} \times 100$$

Assume that the work rate = 600 kpm/min; the estimated VO_2 = 1.47 1 O_2/min (see Reference 16). Then

$$Ew = \frac{(600\ kpm/min)\ (.00234\ kcal/kpm)}{(1.47\ 1\ O_2/min)\ (5.05\ kcal/1\ O_2)} \times 100 = 19\%$$

The above determination of Ew reflects the "gross efficiency" of the body. In general, gross efficiency approximates 20 percent.[12] Since a considerable amount of energy expended by the body is being used merely to maintain life, the measured gross efficiency does not fairly present the true efficiency of the cardiopulmonary and musculoskeletal systems. To determine the "net efficiency" of the working body, the energy required for the maintenance of the body at rest should be deducted from the total energy expenditure. When this is done, Ew is 25 to 30 percent.[12, 13] The remaining 70 to 75 percent unused energy is dissipated from the body as heat energy. With these factors considered, experimentation has shown that the energy cost conversion for mechanical work is slightly less than two milliliters of oxygen per kilogram meter of work (1 kgm $\cong$ 1.8 ml O_2).

Efficiency is related to the intensity and duration of the work. Submaximal aerobic exercise is more efficient than higher intensity anaerobic exercise. One can endure up to 30 to 40 percent of his/her maximal aerobic capacity for an 8-hour working day.[12] Prolonged work at intensities above this level will result in muscular inefficiency and symptoms of exhaustion and fatigue. Patients who have low energy reserves should be advised against doing unnecessary, less efficient, high intensity exercises other than for exercise training purposes. During occupational patient consultations, work load should be considered relative to the patient's aerobic capacity and not just in terms of absolute values, $\dot{V}O_2$ or kcal/min.[3]

ASSESSMENT OF AEROBIC CAPACITY

Physiological Basis and Interpretation

The basic physiological response to exercise is an increase in the total body oxygen consumption. The physiological basis for this response is illustrated by the Fick formula for oxygen uptake ($\dot{V}O_2$):

$$\dot{V}O_2 = \frac{HR \cdot SV}{\dot{Q}} \cdot (a - \bar{v}O_2)$$

The increased oxygen demand during exercise is met by an elevated cardiac output ($\dot{Q}$) as well as an increase in the arteriovenous oxygen difference ($a-\bar{v}O_2$). Greater cardiac output is the result primarily of accelerated heart rate (HR) and, to a lesser extent, greater stroke volume (SV). The increased arteriovenous oxygen difference is the result of an increase in pulmonary ventilation as well as a greater oxygen extraction by the active tissue.

With most types of muscular exercise, steady state oxygen uptake increases linearly with increases in work load to some maximal level referred to as the maximal oxygen uptake ($\dot{V}O_2$ max) or maximal aerobic power (MAP) (Fig. 2-1). Blood lactate progressively increases at the higher exercise intensities and may also be used as a criterion for determining MAP. The maximal work output at $\dot{V}O_2$ max or MAP is referred to as the individual's physical work capacity (PWC) (Fig. 2-1).[12]

In the clinical setting, abnormal or pathological responses to exercise (see Ch. 1) may limit the patient's PWC and prevent the determination of his/her true MAP. The observed maximal exercise capacity in such cases may be referred to as the individual's symptom limited work capacity (SLWC). The term functional aerobic power (FAP) is used to designate the corresponding clinical maximal oxygen uptake.

MAP may be expressed in absolute terms such as liters of oxygen consumed per minute (l O_2/min). Because of the high correlation between the absolute values of MAP and body weight, MAP is also expressed in relative terms normalized to body weight in terms such as milliliters per kilogram of body weight per minute (ml $O_2 \cdot kg^{-1} \cdot min^{-1}$). The latter expression facilitates intersubject comparisons of persons of different body weight and is the accepted unit of measurement when used as an index of cardiovascular function.

A useful clinical method of expressing oxygen uptake is in terms of metabolic equivalents (METs) where one MET is the average oxygen consumption at rest (3.5 ml $O_2 \cdot kg^{-1} \cdot min^{-1}$). This method is commonly used to determine the relative energy cost of a specific work load of an exercise test or of a given physical activity:[17]

$$\text{Relative Oxygen Cost (METs)} = \frac{O_2 \text{ required for work or exercise (ml } O_2 \cdot kg^{-1} \cdot min^{-1})}{O_2 \text{ required at rest (3.5 ml } O_2 \cdot kg^{-1} \cdot min^{-1})}$$

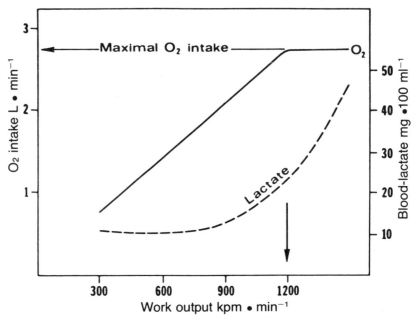

Fig. 2-1. Principle for the direct determination of maximal oxygen intake. Steady state values for oxygen intake are measured at increasing submaximal workloads, and the level established at which a further increase in work rate does not result in any increase in oxygen intake. Note the increase in blood lactate at progressively higher loading. (From Lange-Anderson: Determinants of physical performance capacity in health and disease. In: Exercise Testing and Exercise Training in Coronary Heart Disease, eds. Naughton JP and Hellerstein HK. New York, Academic Press, 1973, by permission).

MAP is an important point of reference in exercise physiology. Individual measurements are highly reproducible and serve as meaningful comprehensive indices of cardiorespiratory fitness and the aerobic capacity of the working muscles.

Differences in body size, age, sex, and habitual level of physical activity account for much of the intersubject variation in MAP.[6, 12] The relationship between MAP and body weight as previously discussed indicates that MAP when expressed in absolute terms will parallel existing variations in body size or stature. MAP increases with age up to 20 years. Beyond this age there is a gradual decline, with an approximate 30 percent deficit by age 60 years. Parallel decreases in maximal heart rate and cardiac output with advancing age may help explain this deficit. Difference in muscle mass accounts for the approximate 15 to 20 percent postpuberty sex difference in MAP. MAP can be increased with physical conditioning (aerobic exercise training); cardiac or pulmonary disease as well as general illness, secondary to physical deconditioning, will produce deficits.

Evaluation of MAP or FAP values is usually based on comparisons with established normative data. Regression equations are available for the prediction of MAP based on age, sex, and habitual level of physical activity (Table 2-2).[18] For

Table 2-2. Prediction of maximal aerobic power

Activity Status[a]	Sex		Predicted MAP (ml O$_2$ · kg^{-1} · min^{-1}[b]
Sedentary	men	=	57.8 − .455 (years of age)
Active	men	=	69.7 − .612 (years of age)
Sedentary	women	=	42.3 − .356 (years of age)
Active	women	=	42.9 − .312 (years of age)

Regression Equations

[a] Persons who do not engage in an aerobic type activity of adequate intensity and duration to develop sweating at least once a week regularly are considered sedentary.

[b] To convert (ml O$_2$·kg^{-1}·min^{-1}) to METs divide by 3.5. (From Bruce RA: Exercise testing of patients with coronary heart disease. Ann Clin Res 3:323–332, 1971)

general reference purposes the ranges of MAP or FAP for cardiac as well as normal subject groups are presented in Table 2-3.[19] MAP values have been classified according to level of cardiorespiratory fitness (Table 2-4).[16] A more definitive method of interpreting MAP or FAP values is based on the determination of functional aerobic impairment (FAI).[18] FAI represents the percent difference between the maximal predicted and observed aerobic power values:

$$FAI = \frac{\text{Predicted Aerobic Power} - \text{Observed Aerobic Power}}{\text{Predicted Aerobic Power}} \times 100$$

Predicted aerobic power is based on the regression equations presented in Table 2-2. A classification scheme for the severity of FAI has been developed and is presented in Table 2-5.[18]

Exercise Testing

Standardized exercise tests have been developed for determining MAP. Detailed descriptions of the currently popular tests are readily available[8, 15, 16] and will not be described in detail here. Only the general characteristics will be considered.

Table 2-3. Maximal/functional aerobic power related to clinical status

Status	mlO$_2$·kg^{-1}·min^{-1}	METs
Symptomatic Patients	3.5–24.5	1–7
Diseased Recovered	7.0–24.5	2–7
Sedentary Healthy	14.0–35.0	4–10
Active Healthy	17.5–56.0	5–16

(From Fox SM, Naughton JP, Haskell WL: Physical activity and the prevention of coronary disease. Ann Clin Res 3: 404–432, 1971)

Table 2-4. Cardiorespiratory fitness classification

| | **Men** | | | | |
| | **Maximal Oxygen Uptake (METs)** | | | | |
Age (yrs)	Low	Fair	Average	Good	High
20–29	<7.2	7.2–9.4	9.5–12.0	12.1–14.8	14.9+
30–39	<6.6	6.6–8.5	8.6–10.8	10.9–13.7	13.8+
40–49	<5.7	5.7–7.4	7.5–10.0	10.1–12.6	12.7+
50–59	<5.1	5.1–6.8	6.9– 9.4	9.5–12.0	12.1+
60–69	<4.6	4.6–6.3	6.4– 8.6	8.7–11.4	11.5+
	Women				
	Maximal Oxygen Uptake (METs)				
Age (yrs)	Low	Fair	Average	Good	High
20–29	<6.8	6.8–8.5	8.6–10.6	10.7–13.7	13.8+
30–39	<5.7	5.7–7.7	7.8– 9.4	9.5–12.6	12.7+
40–49	<4.9	4.9–6.6	6.7– 8.6	8.7–11.7	11.8+
50–59	<4.3	4.3–5.7	5.8– 7.7	7.8–10.6	10.7+
60–69	<3.7	3.7–4.9	5.0– 6.6	6.7– 9.7	9.8+

(Modified from Exercise Testing and Training of Apparently Healthy Individuals: A Handbook for Physicians. p. 15. Dallas, American Heart Association, 1972)

There are basically two types of dynamic exercise tests, the submaximal test and the maximal test. Submaximal tests may consist of one exercise level or of several increasing or graded exercise bouts (single versus multistage tests), and may be performed with or without intervening rest periods (intermittent versus continuous test protocols). The continuous multistage or graded exercise test (GXT) is the most common clinically employed exercise test (see Ch. 6).

The submaximal test is characterized by always having some predetermined arbitrary end point. The end point may be defined in terms of the work load, duration of the exercise, heart rate, or level of oxygen uptake. The usual end point for clinical submaximal exercise tests is a certain percentage of the age predicted maximal heart rate (PMHR); i.e., 85 or 90 percent of PMHR. Maximal heart rate may be predicted from published tables[16] or from the formula: PMHR = 220 − age (years).[19] The submaximal test does not permit direct determinations of MAP. Indirect determination of MAP is based on the linear relationship between steady state submaximal $\dot{V}O_2$ and HR data (Fig. 2-2). MAP is estimated from the end point of the $\dot{V}O_2$ versus HR exercise response curve which is determined by ex-

Table 2-5. Classification of functional aerobic impairment

Severity	% FAI
Mild	27–40
Moderate	41–54
Marked	55–68
Extreme	>69

(From Bruce RA: Exercise testing of patients with coronary heart disease. Ann Clin Res 3: 323–332, 1971)

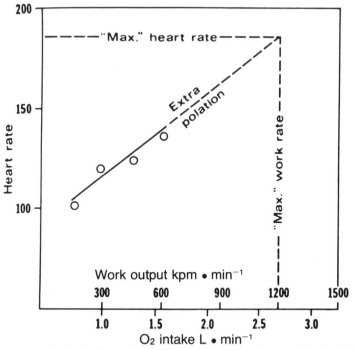

Fig. 2-2. Principle for the indirect determination of maximal oxygen intake. Submaximal heart rates are determined, the linear relationship between heart rate and oxygen intake or work rate established with subsequent extrapolation to the maximal heart rate. (From Lange-Anderson: Determinants of physical performance capacity in health and disease. In: Exercise Testing and Exercise Training in Coronary Heart Disease, eds. Naughton JP and Hellerstein HK. New York, Academic Press, 1973, by permission).

trapolating the line out to the PMHR. Because of the linear relationship between steady state $\dot{V}O_2$ and work load (Fig. 2-1), $\dot{V}O_2$ can be estimated from the standardized work load setting of the exercise testing ergometer. This is the typical clinical approach, since it eliminates the need for collecting, measuring, and analyzing expired air for $\dot{V}O_2$ measurement.

The maximal exercise test is similar in protocol to the submaximal test, but no arbitrary fixed end point other than the individually determined limit of maximal possible or tolerated exertion is used. In contrast to the submaximal test, MAP is determined directly from the achieved work rate. Again, $\dot{V}O_2$ may be determined through actual measurement procedures, or it may be estimated from the achieved work rate.

If the submaximal or maximal tests are terminated because of abnormal exercise response, by the subject, the test is considered to be a symptom limited test with FAP being the outcome.

Selection of exercise intensity and test duration are basic considerations of the GXT. The test must begin with a work load low enough to be submaximal even for subjects with poor physical fitness status. Obviously, the relative exercise intensity will determine the number of exercise bouts and the length of the test. Tests of too short duration will lack sufficient discriminating value while tests of too long duration will submit thermoregulatory mechanisms to excessive stress which will interfere with the accurate assessment of MAP. Practical considerations suggest the use of the basal or resting metabolic energy consumption (METs) as the unit by which to gage the energy demands of the specific work loads.

The basic components of the GXT include:

1. *Baseline.* A preliminary rest period should precede the exercise test in order to collect baseline data.

2. *Warm-up.* A 3 to 5 minute accommodation period should precede the exercise test. A low-level work load should be used (4–5 METs for normal subjects, 2–3 METs for patient groups). During the warm-up or physiological adjustment period, such measurements as HR and blood pressure can facilitate identifying the appropriate initial work load and subsequent increments in work loads for the actual test.

3. *Rest.* The warm-up is followed by 2 minutes of rest while physiological measurements continue. The protocol for the remainder of the test is adjusted or cancelled if any signs of exercise intolerance are observed.

4. *Test.* The duration of the test period depends upon the specific test protocol and the PWC of the subject. Approximately 20 minutes are recommended. The test period should consist of at least 3 to 4 stages or exercise bouts lasting 2 to 5 minutes in duration, each sufficient to achieve physiological steady state. Exercise intensity, work rate is systematically increased so that the subject attains the identified end point (85–90 percent of PMHR for submaximal test, a symptom limited maximal level of exercise for the symptom limited test, or the maximal level of exercise tolerated for the maximal test) during the final exercise stage.

5. *Recovery.* Low intensity exercise should be performed for 3 to 5 minutes following the test period to facilitate recovery and cooling down. The patient should also be monitored for at least 3 minutes while comfortably resting in a chair following the cooling down exercise period.

Testing Ergometers and Estimation of Energy Cost

The three most common exercise testing devices employed in conducting the GXT are: (1) the stepping ergometer, (2) the bicycle ergometer, and (3) the motor-driven treadmill. The ergometers allow for standardization of procedures, which is essential for test accuracy, objectivity, and reliability. Estimation of oxygen requirements may be derived from specific formulas or from published energy equivalent tables (see Tables 2-6–2-10).[4, 16, 20]

The stepping ergometer is a relatively inexpensive device which can have steps of fixed or adjustable heights. It is a flexible tool which can be used in the clinical field or in the laboratory setting. The energy cost of exercising on the stepping ergometer may be determined from the following formula or from Table 2-6.[20]

Table 2-6. Metabolic equivalents (METs) of step ergo-meter work

Height		METs	
		Stepping	Frequency
Inches	Centimeters	20/min	30/min
0	0	2.0	2.8
4	10.2	3.4	4.5
8	20.3	4.7	7.0
12	30.5	6.1	9.5
16	40.5	7.1	12.0

(From Physiological measurements and indices. In: Fitness, Health and Work Capacity: International Standards for Assessment, ed. Larson L. New York, Macmillan, 1973)

$$\dot{V}O_2 \text{ (step ergometer)} = (f \times h \times 1.33 \times 1.8) + Ks$$

$\dot{V}O_2 = O_2$ required in ml $O_2 \cdot kg^{-1} \cdot min^{-1}$ (divide by 3.5 ml $O_2 \cdot kg^{-1} \cdot min^{-1}$ to convert to METs); f = stepping rate or number of vertical lifts per minute (f = 20 is recommended for elderly or convalescing patients; f = 30 is recommended for the healthy sedentary patient); h = the height of the step in meters (1 in = 2.54 cm = .0254 m); 1.33 = work involved in the vertical lift plus 1/3 for descending; 1.8 = ml O_2 equivalent of 1 kpm of work for stepping or other exercise; and Ks = constant which equals the energy expenditure requirement for horizontal forward and backward stepping (at f = 20, Ks $\cong$ 7.0 ml $O_2 \cdot kg^{-1} \cdot min^{-1}$; at f = 30, Ks $\cong$ 10.0 ml $O_2 \cdot kg^{-1} \cdot min^{-1}$.

The bicycle ergometer is the most adaptable of the three testing devices. Bicycle ergometers are constructed with either mechanical or electrical braking systems. The mechanically braked ergometers are constant torque devices which require that the subject pedal at a constant rate. The electrically braked ergometers are variable torque devices in which the work load is automatically maintained within a wide range of pedaling rates: i.e., the power requirement is kept constant through an electrical servo-mechanism which accommodates the brake resistance inversely with the pedaling rate. The mechanical work rate for both types of bicycle ergometers is calibrated in kpm · min^{-1} or watts. The energy cost of exercising

Table 2-7. Metabolic equivalents (METs) of bicycle ergometer work loads

Work Load		Mets According to Body Weight (kg)							
Watts	Kpm/min	50	60	70	80	90	100	110	120
25	150	3.0	2.8	2.6	2.5	2.4	2.3	2.2	2.1
50	300	4.6	4.1	3.7	3.4	3.2	3.0	2.9	2.8
75	450	6.1	5.4	4.8	4.4	4.1	3.8	3.6	3.4
100	600	7.7	6.6	5.9	5.4	4.9	4.6	4.3	4.1
125	750	9.2	7.9	7.0	6.3	5.8	5.4	5.0	4.7
150	900	10.8	9.2	8.1	7.3	6.6	6.1	5.7	5.4
175	1050	12.3	10.5	9.2	8.3	7.5	6.9	6.4	6.0
200	1200	13.8	11.8	10.3	9.2	8.4	7.7	7.1	6.6
250	1500	16.9	14.4	12.5	11.1	10.1	9.2	8.5	7.9
300	1800	20.0	16.9	14.7	13.1	11.8	10.8	9.9	9.2

on the bicycle ergometer may be determined from the following formula or from Table 2-7.[20]

$$\dot{V}O_2 \text{ (bicycle ergometer)} = \text{kpm} \cdot \text{min}^{-1} \times 1.8) + \text{Kt}$$

$\dot{V}O_2$ = requirements in ml O_2/min (to normalize to body weight, divide by the subject's body weight (kg); divide by 3.5 ml $O_2 \cdot \text{kg}^{-1} \cdot \text{min}^{-1}$ to convert to METs); kpm/min = calibrated work rate; 1.8 = ml O_2 biological equivalent of 1 kpm of work; and Kt = constant which equals the energy requirement for pedaling without any load (at work rates < 1800 kgm/min, Kt $\cong$ 5.25 ml $O_2 \cdot \text{kg}^{-1} \cdot \text{min}^{-1}$; at work rates $\geq$ 1800 kgm/min, Kt $\cong$ 7.0 ml $O_2 \cdot \text{kg}^{-1} \cdot \text{min}^{-1}$).

The motor-driven treadmill is one of the most versatile but also most expensive testing devices. Walking speed as well as grade (incline) can be varied to regulate work rate. The energy cost of exercising on the treadmill is depicted in the following formula:

$$\dot{V}O_2 \text{ (treadmill)} = O_2 \text{ cost of level walking} + O_2 \text{ cost of the work associated with the vertical climb}$$

Energy cost estimates are best determined from tabular values based on the specific exercise protocol utilized. The two most clinically common protocols are

Table 2-8. Metabolic equivalents (METs) for the Bruce treadmill exercise test

Exercise Stage	Duration (min)	Total Time (min)	Treadmill Speed (mph)	Percent Grade (% incline)	METs
0	3	1	1.7	0	1.5
		2	1.7	0	2.0
		3	1.7	0	2.0
½	3	4	1.7	5	2.6
		5	1.7	5	3.1
		6	1.7	5	3.1
1	3	7	1.7	10	3.4
		8	1.7	10	4.8
		9	1.7	10	5.1
2	3	10	2.5	12	5.7
		11	2.5	12	6.6
		12	2.5	12	7.1
3	3	13	3.4	14	8.0
		14	3.4	14	9.1
		15	3.4	14	10.0
4	3	16	4.2	16	10.6
		17	4.2	16	13.0
		18	4.2	16	14.0
5	3	19	5.0	18	14.3
		20	5.0	18	15.0
		21	5.0	18	15.7
6	3	22	5.5	20	16.6
		23	5.5	20	18.3
		24	5.5	20	18.9

(From Exercise Testing and Training of Apparently Healthy Individuals: A Handbook for Physicians. Dallas, American Heart Association, 1972)

Table 2-9. Metabolic equivalents (METs) for the standard Balke treadmill exercise test[a]

Exercise Stage	Duration (min)	Total Time (min)	Treadmill Speed (mph)	Percent Grade (% incline)	METs
0	2	2	3	0.0	3
1	2	4	3	2.5	4
2	2	6	3	5.0	5
3	2	8	3	7.5	6
4	2	10	3	10.0	7
5	2	12	3	12.5	8
6	2	14	3	15.0	9
7	2	16	3	17.5	10
8	2	18	3	20.0	11
9	2	20	3	22.5	12

[a] Designed for testing healthy normal subjects.
(Modified from Physiological measurements and indices. In: Fitness, Health and Work Capacity: International Standards for Assessment, ed. Larson L. New York, Macmillan, 1973)

probably the multistage Bruce[16] and Balke[16, 19, 20] tests. The primary difference between these protocols concerns the method of regulating work rate. Grade and speed are varied in Bruce's test; speed is kept constant and only grade is varied in Balke's test. The reader should refer to the indicated references and to Chapter 6 for a more complete description of the test protocols. The energy cost estimates according to exercise stage for these two tests are presented in Tables 2-8, 2-9 and 2-10.[16, 19, 20]

ENERGY COST OF PHYSICAL ACTIVITIES

The physical activity component of a comprehensive cardiac rehabilitation program must meet the individual needs of the patient during each stage of recovery. The typical phases included in the cardiac rehabilitation program are: hospitalization, coronary care unit and intermediate coronary care unit; convalescence, outpatient hospital-based or home program; and recovery, long-term community-based or home program.[21, 22]

Table 2-10. Metabolic equivalents (METs) for the substandard Balke treadmill exercise test[a]

Exercise Stage	Duration (min)	Total Time (min)	Treadmill Speed (mph)	Percent Grade (% incline)	METs
1	2	2	2.0	0	2
2	2	4	2.0	2.5	2.66
3	2	6	2.0	5.0	3.33
4	2	8	2.0	7.5	4.00
5	2	10	2.0	10.0	4.66
6	2	12	2.0	12.5	5.33
7	2	14	2.0	15.0	6.00
8	2	16	2.0	17.5	6.66
9	2	18	2.0	20.0	7.33
10	2	20	2.0	22.5	8.00

[a] Designed for testing subjects with pathological cardiorespiratory fitness.
(Modified from Physiological measurements and indices. In: *Fitness, Health and Work Capacity: International Standards for Assessment,* ed. Larson L. New York, Macmillan, 1973)

Early ambulation is emphasized for the cardiac patient during the hospitalization phase to help offset the physiological effects of prolonged bedrest.[23] In coronary artery bypass graft surgery patients, physical activity, including range of motion and breathing exercises as well as ambulation, is used to decrease postsurgical stiffness and prevent/treat postoperative pulmonary complications. While the general focus of the inpatient phases of the program is on maintenance (preventing deconditioning), the emphasis of the outpatient phase is on improvement of physical fitness.

Realistic activity preferences and goals are established by integrating the results of the patient assessment, including the results of the GXT, with information obtained from interviewing the patient, from the medical history of the patient, and from other rehabilitation team members. Guidelines are available for establishing activity and training levels for the cardiac patient (see Ch. 8).[3, 22, 24] Relative exercise intensity and work rate are basic considerations. Heart rate is usually the standard indicator of relative exercise intensity, while energy cost reflects the work rate of the exercise. Energy cost needs to be considered when planning treatment and training programs and when recommending activity levels.

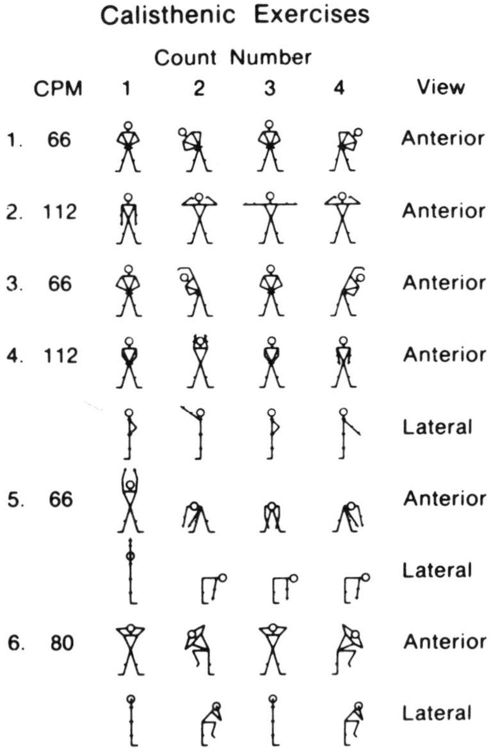

Fig. 2-3. Calisthenic exercises (CPM = counts per minute). (From Amundsen LR, Takahashi M, Carter CA, Nielsen DH: Energy cost of rehabilitation calisthenics. Phys Ther 59:855–858, 1979, by permission).

Table 2-11. Approximate energy requirements of cardiac rehabilitation inpatient phase physical activities[a]

Activity	METs
1. Self-care activities in bed with back supported[26]	
Feeding self	1.5
Washing hands and face	1.5
Washing body while sitting in a chair (excluding back and legs)	1.7
Brushing teeth	1.5
Care of fingernails	1.5
Shaving	1.6
Combing hair	1.6
2. Assisted transfer and use of bedside commode[26]	1.5
3. Physical exercises[26]	
Passive ROM[b] exercises to all extremities	1.0
Active ROM exercises to all extremities	1.0–1.5
Active ROM exercises with moderate resistance to all extremities	1.5–2.0
4. Calisthenic Exercises (see Fig. 2-3)[27]	
Exercise #1	1.7
Exercise #2	2.3
Exercise #3	2.8
Exercise #4	2.9
Exercise #5	5.1
Exercise #6	5.9
5. Ambulation[28]	
0.5 mph (13.4 m/min)	1.8
1.0 mph (26.8 m/min)	1.9
1.5 mph (40.2 m/min)	2.2
2.0 mph (53.6 m/min)	2.5
2.5 mph (67.1 m/min)	3.0
3.0 mph (80.5 m/min)	3.5
3.5 mph (93.9 m/min)	4.1
4.0 mph (107.3 m/min)	4.8

[a] Includes resting metabolic needs.
[b] ROM = range of motion.

Numerous energy cost charts and tables of various physical activities have been published.[1, 6, 12, 16, 25–28] Tables 2-11 and 2-12 and Figure 2-3 have been included to provide a convenient listing of the energy cost of specific physical activities typically considered in cardiac rehabilitation programs.

Table 2-12. Approximate energy requirements of cardiac rehabilitation outpatient phase physical activities[a]

Category	Self-care or Home	Occupational	Recreational[b]	Physical Conditioning
Very light <3 METs	Washing, shaving, dressing Desk work, writing Washing dishes Driving auto	Sitting (clerical, assembling) Standing (store clerk, bartender) Driving truck[b] Crane operator[b]	Shuffleboard Horseshoes Bait casting Billiards Archery[b] Golf (cart)	Walking (level at 2 mph) Stationary bicycle (very lo resistance) Very light calisthenics
Light 3–5 METs	Cleaning windows Raking leaves Weeding Power lawn mowing Waxing floors (slowly) Painting Carrying objects (15–30 lb)	Stocking shelves (light objects) Light welding Light carpentry[c] Machine assembly Auto repair Paper hanging[c]	Dancing (social and square) Golf (walking) Sailing Horseback riding Volleyball (6 man) Tennis (doubles)	Walking (3–4 mph) Level bicycling (6–8 mph) Light calisthenics
Moderate 5–7 METs	Easy digging in garden Level hand lawn mowing Climbing stairs (slowly) Carrying objects (30–60 lb)[c]	Carpenty (exterior home building)[c] Shoveling dirt[c] Pneumatic tools[c]	Badminton (competitive) Tennis (singles) Snow skiing (downhill) Light backpacking Basketball Football Skating (ice and roller) Horseback riding (gallop)	Walking (4.5–5 mph) Bicycling (9–10 mph) Swimming (breast stroke)
Heavy 7–9 METs	Sawing wood[c] Heavy shoveling[c] Climbing stairs (moderate speed) Carrying objects (60–90 lb)[c]	Tending furnace[c] Digging ditches[c] Pick and shovel[c]	Canoeing[c] Mountain climbing[c] Fencing Paddleball Touch football	Jog (5 mph) Swim (crawl stroke) Rowing machine Heavy calisthenics Bicycling (12 mph)
Very heavy >9 METs	Carrying loads upstairs[c] Carrying objects (>90 lb)[c] Climbing stairs (quickly) Shoveling heavy snow[c] Shoveling 10/min (16 lb)	Lumberjack[c] Heavy laborer[c]	Handball Squash Ski touring over hills[c] Vigorous basketball	Running (≥6 mph) Bicycle (≥13 mph or up steep hill) Rope jumping

[a] Includes resting metabolic needs.
[b] May cause added psychologic stress that will increase work load on the heart.
[c] May produce disproportionate myocardial demands because of use of arms or isometric exercise.
(Modified from Haskell WL: Design and implementation of cardiac conditioning programs. In: Rehabilitation of the Coronary Patient, eds. Wenger NK, Hellerstein HK. New York, John Wiley and Sons, 1978)

REFERENCES

1. Fox SM, Naughton JP, Gorman PA: Physical activity and cardiovascular health. Mod Concepts Cardiovasc Dis 41:17–30, 1972
2. Report of Inter-Society Commission for Heart Disease Resources: Primary Prevention of the Atherosclerotic Diseases. Circulation 42:A-55–A-95, December 1970
3. Amundsen LR: Establishing activity and training levels for patients with ischemic heart disease. Phys Ther 59:754–758, 1979
4. Naughton JP, Hellerstein HK, Mohler IC, eds.: Exercise Testing and Training in Coronary Heart Disease. New York, Academic Press, 1973
5. Zohman LR, Tobis JS: Cardiac Rehabilitation. New York, Grune and Stratton, 1970
6. Haskell WL: Design and implementation of cardiac conditioning programs. In: Rehabilitation of the Coronary Patient, eds. Wenger NK, Hellerstein HK. New York, John Wiley and Sons, 1978
7. Rose G: Early mobilization and discharge after myocardial infarction. Mod Concepts Cardiovasc Dis 41:59–63, 1972
8. Johnston BL, Cantwell JD, Fletcher GF: Rehabilitation of the critically ill: eight steps to inpatient cardiac rehabilitation: the team effort-methodology and preliminary results. Heart Lung 5:97–111, 1976
9. Grant A, Cohen BS: Acute myocardial infarction: effect of rehabilitation program on length of hospitalization and functional status at discharge. Arch Phys Med Rehabil 54:201–206, 1973
10. Lehninger, AL: Biochemistry. New York, Worth Publishers, 1970
11. Needham D: Machina Carnis: The Biochemistry of Muscular Contraction in Its Historical Development. New York, Cambridge University Press, 1971
12. Åstrand P-O, Rodahl K: Textbook of Work Physiology, New York, McGraw Hill, 1977
13. Wasserman K, Whipp BJ: State of the art: exercise physiology in health and disease. Am Rev Respir Dis (112):219–249, 1975
14. Blomquist CG: Clinical exercise physiology. In: Rehabilitation of the Coronary Patient, eds. Wenger NK, Hellerstein HK. New York, John Wiley and Sons, 1978
15. Wasserman K, Whipp BJ, Koyal SN, Beaver WL: Anaerobic threshold and respiratory gas exchange during exercise. J Appl Physiol 35:236–243, 1973
16. Exercise Testing and Training of Apparently Healthy Individuals: A Handbook for Physicians. Dallas, American Heart Association, 1972
17. Exercise Testing and Training of Individuals with Heart Disease or at High Risk for Its Development: A Handbook for Physicians. Dallas, American Heart Association, 1975
18. Bruce RA: Exercise testing of patients with coronary heart disease. Ann Clin Res 3:323–332, 1971
19. Fox SM, Naughton JP, Haskell WL: Physical activity and the prevention of coronary disease. Ann Clin Res 3:404–432, 1971
20. Physiological measurements and indices. In: Fitness, Health and Work Capacity: International Standards for Assessment, ed. Larson L. New York, Macmillan, 1973
21. Pollock ML, Ward A, Foster C: Prescriptions of exercise in cardiac rehabilitation program. In: Cardiac Rehabilitation Implications for the Nurse and Other Health Professionals, eds. Fardy PS, Bennett, JL, Reitz NL, Williams MA. St. Louis, CV Mosby, 1980

22. Saltin B, Blomquist G, Mitchell JH, et al: Response to exercise after bedrest and after training. Circulation 38 (suppl 7): entire issue, 1968
23. Naughton JP: The contribution of regular physical activity to the ambulatory care of cardiac patients. Postgrad Med 57:51–55, 1975
24. Cunningham DA, Rechnitzer PA: Exercise prescription and the postcoronary patient. Arch Phys Med Rehabil 55:276–300, 1977
25. Meyer GC: Exercises for the inpatient. Cardiac Rehabilitation Implications for the Nurse and Other Health Professionals, eds Fardy PS, Bennett JL, Reitz NL, Williams MA. St. Louis, CV Mosby, 1980
26. Activities Which Require a MET Level in the Cardiac Rehabilitation Program. Department of Physical Medicine, St. Joseph Mercy Hospital, Ann Arbor, MI, 1972
27. Amundsen LR, Takahashi M, Carter CA, Nielsen DH: Energy cost of rehabilitation calisthenics. Phys Ther 59:855–858, 1979
28. Rohrig WL: Submaximal Exercise Testing: Treadmill and Floor Walking. Master's Thesis, University of Iowa, Programs in Physical Therapy, 1978

3 | Physiological Effects of Endurance Training

Theresa Hoskins Michel

DEFINITION OF ENDURANCE TRAINING

Endurance training may be carried out by athletes, by healthy individuals who do not aspire to competitive sports, and by convalescents from vascular and other debilitating diseases. The goals of these different classes of individuals are of necessity very different, although all strive for an improvement in physical fitness and functional capacity. The athlete trains at an intensity designed to exact his maximal performance. The healthy middle-aged worker engages in a modest training program to achieve fitness, and the convalescent, who probably starts at a low initial level of fitness, may perform at very low intensities and yet produce a relatively large increase in physical working capacity.

All of these individuals, aiming for improved fitness, will concentrate on aerobic exercise. Isometric exercises, which are useful for increasing muscular strength and muscle mass, rely on anaerobic metabolism, and will contribute to an improvement in anaerobic work capacity, or improved ability to tolerate an oxygen debt. Aerobic exercise involves submaximal, dynamic exercise of longer than several minutes duration, using large muscle groups. It is the aerobic form of exercise which contributes to the improvement of all parts of the oxygen transport system, and especially to the cardiovascular system.[1]

During dynamic exercise, the large demand for oxygen by working muscle is met by large increases in stroke volume and heart rate, with a marked reduction of peripheral vascular resistance. This combination produces high cardiac outputs (heart rate × stroke volume) and very little alteration in mean arterial blood pressure. The high cardiac output results in elevated systolic blood pressures, but the low peripheral resistance often drops the diastolic blood pressure readings.

29

Thus, this type of cardiac work is referred to as volume loading of the left ventricle.

Static or isometric exercise produces extremely large increases in mean, systolic, and diastolic arterial pressures even with a small mass of skeletal muscle contracting. At the same time, there are relatively small increases in heart rate and cardiac output. Stroke volume and peripheral vascular resistance remain unchanged. This type of contraction therefore results in a pressure load on the left ventricle.

The potential benefits of dynamic, aerobic exercise over an adequate training period to the cardiovascular system are those which should promote a more efficient system better adapted to higher physical work levels, and perhaps beneficial to the health and function of individuals who have myocardial impairment. The evidence for this is presented in this chapter.

EFFECTS OF ENDURANCE TRAINING IN NORMAL INDIVIDUALS

Endurance training significantly improves the oxygen transport capabilities of the human organism. Oxygen transport ultimately determines an individual's maximal physical working capacity and is a total system of many component parts. Not all of these parts respond equally favorably to endurance training, yet many parts are altered, made more efficient, or in some way improved. Since the process of delivering oxygen to working muscle, where it ultimately is used for metabolism, involves a step-ladder of progression through the various organ systems, it may be useful to follow the oxygen molecule's progress down the ladder of the oxygen transport system.

Pulmonary System

The muscles of ventilation are responsible for beginning the molecule's travels. Oxygen must be pulled into the body from the surrounding air, which is done by creating a suction at the nose and mouth with each inspiration. Since the inside of the lung is a negative pressure with respect to the atmospheric pressure, the more negative this pressure becomes through more forceful and larger inspirations, the stronger the suction force created. Oxygen molecules inside the lung travel in the bronchioles to the alveoli, where the capillary-to-alveolar membrane is encountered.

Endurance exercise does not influence the muscles of ventilation in the normal person who has no lung disease or unusual muscle weakness. The measured alveolar ventilations during maximal exercise rarely equal the maximal voluntary ventilation levels generated at rest, but in the highly trained endurance athlete, the maximal exercise alveolar ventilation is closer to the maximal voluntary ventilation measured at rest. In many cases there is an increase in lung volume and vital capacity after training.[2] These changes allow the trained individual to deliver more oxygen to the alveoli during maximal effort.

Next the oxygen molecule traverses the alveolar membrane to enter the bloodstream and attach to a hemoglobin molecule. This is done by a passive process of diffusion and is sped up by higher oxygen partial pressures and by high concentrations of hemoglobin ready for bonding. It has been shown that alveolar diffusion is enhanced in the trained individual, perhaps due to higher hemoglobin concentrations, or to some factors relating to the membrane itself.[2] During exercise, the end-diastolic and peak systolic pressures of the right ventricle and the hydrostatic pressure of the lung capillaries are higher in trained subjects.[3] Thus, more driving force is behind the blood entering the lungs to be oxygenated, permitting a faster diffusion of oxygen as hemoglobin is made more available.

Circulatory System

Once bonded with hemoglobin, the oxyhemoglobin molecular complex travels from lung capillaries into the pulmonary veins draining the lungs and returns to the left atrium of the heart. Here, the oxygenated blood must pass through the mitral valve into the left ventricle. Efficient passage depends upon the integrity of the large cusped valve and the relative pressure differential between the low pressure atrium and the thick walled left ventricle. The adequate function of this valve is vital to the proper transfer of oxygenated blood from the atrium to the ventricle.

The left ventricle is the next vital component in the transport of this oxyhemoglobin molecular complex. This ventricle is responsible for the forceful expulsion of blood out the aorta and to all organs of the body requiring oxygenated blood. It acts as a pump and, as such, has two mechanisms by which it can pump more blood per unit of time to meet higher exercise demands. One mechanism is to pump faster via an increase in heart rate, and the other is to pump more volume of blood with each contraction, either by permitting more blood to enter the chamber prior to forcing it out, or by a stronger force of contraction, squeezing out more of the blood contained within the chamber. Endurance training usually has a major effect on the function of the left ventricle.

Endurance training lowers the resting heart rate and the exercise heart rate at submaximal levels of exertion, and usually has no effect on maximal heart rate in normal individuals. This effect seems contrary to the desirable effect of pumping more blood per unit of time. However, this lowering of heart rate benefits the heart by decreasing myocardial oxygen cost, and as long as the stroke volume increases, cardiac output can be maintained. Also the lower heart rate at each submaximal exercise load permits a more gradual rise in heart rate to maximum, with higher intensities of exercise possible without increasing maximal heart rate. Since, in fact, the cardiac output stays roughly the same before and after endurance training and the heart rate is lower at equivalent work rates, the stroke volume therefore has risen to compensate for lower heart rates.[3] The mechanism of the higher stroke volumes is not clearly defined. With greater venous return, there would be higher diastolic volumes, more stretch on the heart muscle, and a greater force of contraction (Frank-Starling Mechanism) as well as greater volumes of blood available for each ventricular contraction. These factors may increase with endurance training. The most significant mechanism for increasing stroke volume is due to the inotropic effects of sympathetic nerve stimulation enhancing the contractility of the myocardium.[4]

The next consideration for the transport of the oxygen molecule is the regional distribution of blood flow. Optimally, more blood will be delivered to areas of highest need: the exercising muscles, the heart itself, and the brain: and less blood will be distributed to the splanchnic, renal, and non-exercising muscle regions. This clearly is optimized by endurance training in normal individuals.[5] If there is a higher capillary flow in exercising muscle, then there is greater contact of the oxygen molecule with the working muscle cells, which aids in the transfer of oxygen across the capillary membrane.[6]

Muscle Metabolism

Skeletal muscle metabolic machinery is located in the mitochondria and consists of two possible energy pathways: aerobic when oxygen is present, and anaerobic when oxygen is not present or is insufficient for the exercise demand. When the oxyhemoglobin molecule arrives at an arteriovenous capillary of a contracting skeletal muscle, the oxygen will be dissociated from its hemoglobin and used in the mitochondria in the final stages of the Kreb's oxidative cycle as the final electron receptor. Without oxygen, the Kreb's cycle is backed up, and the anaerobic glycolysis cycle begins producing energy plus lactate as a by-product. The differences between these two cycles are many, but of major functional significance is the fact that there is a much higher energy yield for each molecule of fuel substrate (carbohydrate, fat, or protein) when oxygen is available. Individuals performing aerobic activities can truly endure much longer efforts than those performing anaerobic activities. Thus, "endurance training" is synonymous with aerobic training.

Aerobic training has been shown to increase the number of mitochondria in muscle cells, and there is a concurrent rise in the activity of the enzymes involved in the Kreb's cycle.[7] In addition, the proportionate volume of red muscle fibers, which are capable of storing oxygen in the form of myoglobin, increase, while white fibers, which are adapted to anaerobic metabolism, are proportionately less.[8] These muscular and metabolic adaptations to training account for a measurable increase in the arteriovenous oxygen difference at the capillary exchange step in the ladder. Thus, there is a greater unloading of oxygen by hemoglobin because of a higher capacity to use oxygen by the muscle cells, and the difference in oxygen content of the venous side to the arterial side of the capillary bed is greater. This represents the final rung of the ladder for the oxygen molecule, because once it combines with its final electron, it becomes carbon dioxide and reverses the direction of movement to be eliminated by the lungs in exchange for a new oxygen molecule.

Additional Effects

In addition to an enhancement of the oxygen transport system, many other effects of endurance training have been investigated in normal individuals. Endocrine effects have been documented: a reduction in catecholamine rise during exercise may transfer to other situations to contribute to higher tolerance for stress, both physical and mental.[9] Training leads to an increase in parasympathetic dominance at rest.[10] Psychological effects have been studied. In general, all subjects report subjective experiences of more contentment and less tension in life.[11]

Muscle strength and endurance increase with endurance training, but only in the muscles actively engaged in the training.[12] The heart muscle undergoes hypertrophy with endurance training and becomes a stronger muscle pump.[13]

People who train in hot climates become acclimatized to heat faster than sedentary people moving to hot climates.[14] Even in regular climates, training seems to promote an optimum temperature regulation of the body, with more efficient sweating for unloading heat. The central nervous system benefits from endurance training. Faster reaction times, better coordination, and more accuracy of movement have been recorded.[15]

Blood elements may shift with training. There is an increase in fibrinolysis.[16] Serum triglycerides are reduced 2 hours after an exercise session, and this reduction lasts 2 to 3 days.[17] There is better utilization of free fatty acids in peripheral muscles, and a trained subject has less ketones and lower increases in pyruvate and lactate during exercise.[18] Endurance training increases the ratio of high density lipoproteins to low density and very low density lipoproteins. Lipoproteins are the carrier molecules for cholesterol. The shift to higher high density lipoproteins is associated with reduction in risk for coronary heart disease.[19]

Does endurance training of normal apparently healthy individuals reduce the risk for coronary heart disease, both myocardial infarction and mortality? This question has not been conclusively answered. Studies investigating the role of exercise training in primary prevention have been fraught with difficulties. People with risk factors engage in multiple intervention programs, and the role of exercise cannot be isolated. Few studies have used control groups, and those that have, often have selection bias due to using drop-outs for non-exercising controls. These same problems have plagued studies on secondary prevention as well. The controversy continues to rage, with strong supporters of exercise exaggerating the benefits, and antagonists to exercise finding reasons to remain sedentary.

EFFECTS OF ENDURANCE TRAINING IN PATIENTS WITH CORONARY ARTERY DISEASE

Alterations Imposed by the Disease

The physiologic mechanisms of adaptation in asymptomatic, apparently healthy control subjects who undergo endurance training have been studied extensively, and many are well understood. In cases in which coronary blood flow is impaired and ventricular wall mechanics have been altered by myocardial infarction, entirely new studies must be done to measure the increase in variability in the physiologic responses to both acute exercise and endurance training. Some studies have been conducted but many more are needed.

Some of the alterations in heart function imposed by ischemic heart disease include reductions in stroke volume, but near normal cardiac output at rest and at submaximal levels of exercise, and reductions in maximal heart rate. Maximal cardiac outputs are therefore limited.[20] An increase in heart rate compensates for the reduction in stroke volume at rest and at low levels of exercise. However, the decreased capacity to raise the heart rate and stroke volume causes the maximal physical work rates possible for these patients to be less than normal.

Why is the stroke volume reduced in patients with coronary artery disease? Probably this is due to a diminished ability of the left ventricle to contract during systole, with a resulting reduction in the ejection fraction. Ejection fraction refers to the amount of blood ejected with each contraction (systole). Normally, this is about 70 percent of the blood inside the ventricle at the end of the diastolic filling period. The ejection fraction is calculated as the ratio of stroke volume to the end-diastolic volume. During upright exercise in the normal heart, the end-systolic volume decreases (more blood is ejected) and the end-diastolic volume increases (more venous return and more filling volume, and greater stretch applied to the ventricle). In patients with coronary heart disease, there may be an increase in end-systolic volume (less blood is ejected due to the weakened muscle), resulting in a lowering of the ejection fraction.[21]

Why is the maximal heart rate limited in patients? It is possible that the abnormal wall motion in patients who are post-myocardial infarction results in activation of ventricular mechanoreceptors which reflexly cause bradycardia and peripheral vasodilation.[22] Relative ischemia of the SA node will also reduce maximal heart rates.

Cardiac patients demonstrate improvements in physical working capacity just as normal subjects do. The mechanisms of their improvement may or may not be identical to those defined for asymptomatic, apparently healthy individuals. Various studies using a variety of techniques have been employed, ranging from sophisticated measures of cardiac output or of coronary vessel size and collateralization during coronary angiography to relatively simple stress testing procedures and indirect indices of cardiac function. Maximal oxygen consumption increases in patients after an appropriate period of endurance training at sufficient intensities and frequencies (see Fig. 3-1).[10, 23] Since this measure is the best single index of the total oxygen transport system, we can conclude that mechanisms of improvement in oxygen transport for patients may be similar to those evaluated in normals.

Pulmonary System

Cardiac patients who do not have concomitant lung disease, or who have no active congestive heart failure, do not differ in their training response from normal individuals. However, they do often experience dyspnea at some high effort

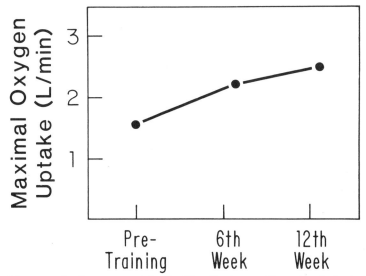

Fig. 3-1. Mean maximal oxygen uptake for 18 patients over 12 weeks of physical training.

level, and training seems to improve their ability to exercise longer at higher intensities, before experiencing dyspnea. Dyspnea is a poorly understood symptom, and the mechanism of improvement is not clear. However, as patients become trained, they achieve higher maximal ventilations, and at each submaximal level, ventilation is achieved by the more efficient mechanism of lower respiratory rates and higher tidal volumes.[1]

Circulatory System

Endurance training does not usually improve the cardiac output in coronary artery disease, but the same hemodynamic alterations seen in normals are also obvious in this group. The heart rate is significantly lower at each submaximal work load, which means the stroke volume is greater after training than before. The maximal heart rate usually increases slightly (see Fig. 3-2).[10] This alteration produces a more efficient muscle pump, even though in the case of post-myocardial infarction patients, the muscle has an area of scar and possible hypokinesis.[24]

Another well documented effect of endurance training in the cardiac patient is a lowered resting blood pressure.[25] In many patients, the systolic blood pressure is consistently lower at each submaximal work load as well. Since the product of the heart rate and the systolic blood pressure is useful in the estimation of myocardial function, it is often used as an important non-invasive measure of improvement. The rate-pressure product (RPP) is significant because it has a high correlation ($r=0.90$) with myocardial oxygen consumption.[26, 27] A high RPP at any level of work indicates an inefficient cardiovascular system which is causing the heart to make greater effort at more O_2 cost to meet the demands of the workload. This inefficient system cannot increase the cardiac output very much in spite

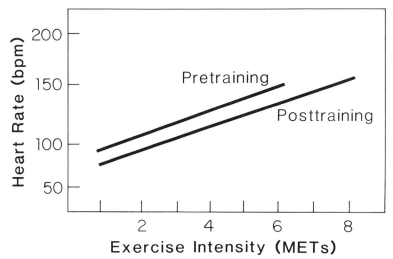

Fig. 3-2.   Effect of training on heart rate response of cardiac patients.

of large increases in systolic blood pressures. Large increases in systolic blood pressure with small increases in cardiac output reflect an inability of the poorly conditioned cardiovascular system to adequately decrease the total peripheral resistance. Since conditioning patients does reduce RPP, there is an improvement in myocardial efficiency, and in the ability to decrease total peripheral resistance (see Fig. 3-3).[10, 23]

At maximal effort, which after training reaches a new higher work rate, conditioning often results in an increase in maximal RPP, indicating an increased power output of the heart, and an increase in myocardial oxygen consumption (see Fig. 3-3). In cardiac patients who are symptomatic, this finding is very signifi-

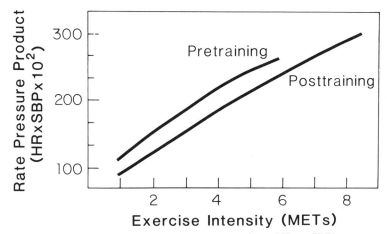

Fig. 3-3.   Effect of training on mean rate-pressure product (HR × SBP) responses of cardiac patients.

cant. The heart can now tolerate more work before symptoms of angina or isch-emic changes on the EKG appear. How can it do this? Several potential mecha-nisms have been proposed. There may be an increase in myocardial oxygen sup-ply, thus permitting more oxygen consumption by the myocardium. There may be a decrease in the oxygen demands of the myocardium at any given level of work, or there may be less myocardial work for an equal cardiac output. Studies to de-termine the answer have inherent difficulties, and results remain inconclusive. To study myocardial oxygen supply requires invasive measures done before and after training, and in the treatment as well as in a control group of coronary heart dis-eased patients. It has not always been possible to recruit control or comparison groups, and there are several confounding influences, such as the natural progression of the disease, and the possibility of spontaneous improvement in car-diovascular responses to exercise even without training.

Five mechanisms for increasing myocardial oxygen supply have been stud-ied: (1) retrogression or delay of progression of coronary atherosclerosis, (2) in-crease in lumen diameter of major coronary vessels, (3) coronary collateral vascu-larization, (4) redistribution of regional blood flow, and (5) increase in volume of blood flowing to an ischemic area.

Several studies investigated the first of these mechanisms. In the early stud-ies, no control groups were used, and in the majority of patients studied, there was no progression of disease, as visualized with arteriography before and after one year of training.[28, 29] In a study of four groups of patients, who were self selected for intensity of training, and who worked on the modification of all their risk fac-tors simultaneously, the two groups who trained the hardest had significantly less progression of coronary plaque in the coronary arteries as viewed by arteriogra-phy after 20 months of training. The two groups who were either sedentary, or who engaged in low levels of activity, showed more plaque progression over the same period.[30]

In addition to this direct evidence, some indirect evidence for favorable training effects upon the rate of atherosclerosis has been compiled. The high den-sity lipoprotein fraction of blood increases with training, while the low and very low density lipoprotein fractions decrease. A high level of high density lipoprotein fraction is associated with protection from coronary atherosclerosis.[19] Also in these studies, the rise in high density lipoproteins is more systematic with exercise than with dietary measures of control, or with weight reduction. Exercise training delays blood clotting which may impact upon thrombotic disease in general.[31] Training in cardiac patients increases fibrinolysis significantly.[16] In diabetics and hyperglycemics, training tends to normalize carbohydrate metabolism.

Lumen diameter has been studied, but usually not in the population of post-myocardial infarction patients. Autopsies performed on marathon runners, of all ages and types and with all causes of death, have shown remarkably large lumen diameters of coronary vessels, and few if any signs of occlusion or significant plaque.[32] More often, measures of coronary flow, as an indirect index of lumen size, are obtained in coronary patients.

A number of studies on coronary collateral vascularization have been re-ported, but all of these are on small numbers of patients, and no control subjects are included. The adequate stimulus to produce collateral branching of coronary arteries is myocardial hypoxia, induced by plaques and an imposed increase in myocardial work. The hypothesis that the increase in coronary perfusion pressure or coronary blood flow produced during exercise will result in tissue hypoxia, followed by dilatation and enlargement of small vessels at regions distal to significant lesions, is reasonable, but has never been adequately substantiated by these studies. In one such study, 21 coronary artery occlusions were identified by angiography in 14 patients, but only 2 of these lesions showed new collaterals after 13 months of low-intensity games and walking 3 times per week for 1 hour. Both lesions were progressing to complete or nearly complete stenosis, which may be the critical determinant permitting collateral sprouting.[28] This study included no measure of coronary blood flow, which would help to substantiate the hypothesis. The current state of visualization of coronary collateral vascularization using angiography is admittedly insensitive to smaller vessels, and may not be an adequate measure for this type of study.

Coronary blood flow has been measured using coronary sinus blood flow with thermodilution techniques.[33] A comparison before and after 6 months of endurance training (30 minutes of a stationary bicycle and 20 minutes of volleyball 2.6 times per week for 16–22 weeks) showed that the coronary sinus blood flow was less at rest after training, along with lower heart rates and lower systolic blood pressures. The same relationship held true at low work loads, but at the angina threshold work load, there was a higher coronary sinus blood flow after training but the difference was not significant. Six of 10 patients had a rise in their maximal coronary sinus blood flow following training. This measure clearly does not provide regional blood flow information, nor has there been any development of a suitable measure of volume of blood flowing to ischemic regions, especially microcirculatory measurement techniques.

Since there is no significant evidence for an improvement in myocardial oxygen supply with training, the primary mechanism of improved functional capacity may well lie on the other side of the coin, with a decrease in myocardial oxygen demand taking place with training. The fact that the RPP notably drops with training at each submaximal level of work is good evidence in support of this mechanism. Why training induces bradycardia has been studied by numerous investigators, and many different theories have arisen. Measures include skeletal muscle changes (peripheral) and central blood volume increases,[34] increases in myocardial hypertrophy,[35] increases in myocardial contractility,[12] and altered central nervous system regulation.[36] The conclusions from these studies seem to be that much of the heart rate decrease is due to changes taking place in the active skeletal muscles. In addition, there is a lower sympathetic tone during exercise in trained patients, and at rest, the vagal tone is higher in these patients.[37] Plasma catecholamines have also been measured and are reduced by exercise training in these patients.[9]

The skeletal muscle changes referred to are identical changes to those found in the normal population, and also account for the widening of the arteriovenous oxygen difference, with greater numbers of mitochondria. This permits muscles to function at lower oxygen saturation levels.[38]

Another very beneficial effect of endurance training on patients with myocardial irritability appears to be an antidysrrhythmic potential for some individuals. However, not enough investigations have been performed to substantiate this hypothesis, and there is a need to define what criteria determine this effect.[39]

Psychological Effects of Training in Coronary Patients

Patients subjectively report improvements in their state of mind and sense of well-being, and often report feeling "more normal" again. These changes are difficult to demonstrate on existing psychological tests. The Minnesota Multiphasic Personality Inventory (MMPI) has been used by several investigators. Cardiac patients consistently, as a group, show higher depression and psychasthenia scores than normals, and these scores do decline after a period of training.[40] After 12–15 months of endurance training, ⅓ of the total group of 610 patients in the Toronto Cardiac Rehabilitation Program still showed the neurotic triad: hysteria, hypochondriasis, and psychasthenia, and also showed very high depression scores. After 4 more years of continued training, small gains were made in the MMPI results in the same subjects.[41]

In another study, after 18 months of training, significant improvements in visual speed and ability to concentrate were objectively measured, while subjective responses of reduction in psychic tension and nervousness, and improved ability to relax and to tolerate stress were reported.[15] Other behavioral characteristics which improve with endurance training are more regular eating habits, longer calmer sleep, and a more tranquil attitude to home and work conflicts.[42] In a study using a control group of normal adults who also trained, both groups reported less tension, more contentment.[11]

CONCLUSIONS

It may be that beneficial effects on coronary artery disease have not been adequately demonstrated to convincing degrees, because the studies have been severely hampered by poor compliance, too short a duration of training, inadequate intensity of training, and inadequate measurement of critical parameters. Exercise training may act in its own right in some or all of the mechanisms hypothesized so far, but it may also act indirectly by modifying other risk factors such as body weight, hypertension, serum lipids, and smoking behavior. The majority of patients benefit in intangible ways, and more studies with better controls should be carried out to document any objective benefits training may have on the atherosclerotic disease process itself.

REFERENCES

1. Åstrand P-O, Rodahl K: Textbook of Work Physiology. New York, McGraw-Hill, 1977
2. Grimby G: Respiration in exercise. Med Sci Sports 1:9–14, 1969

3. Bevegård S, Holmgren A, Jonsson B: Circulatory studies in well trained athletes at rest and during heavy exercise, with special reference to stroke volume and the influence of body position. Acta Physiol Scand 57:26, 1963

4. Cardus D, Fuentes F, Scrinivasan R: Cardiac evaluation of a physical rehabilitation program for patients with ischemic heart disease. Arch Phys Med Rehabil 56:419–425, 1975

5. Clausen JP, Trap-Jensen J: Effects of training on the distribution of cardiac output in patients with coronary artery disease. Circulation 42:611–624, 1970

6. Kentala E: Physical fitness and feasibility of physical rehabilitation after myocardial infarction in men of working age. Ann Clin Res 4(Suppl 9):1–84, 1972

7. Holloszy JO: Biochemical adaptations in muscle. Effects of exercise on mitochondrial oxygen uptake and respiratory enzyme activity in skeletal muscle. J Biol Chem 242:2278, 1967

8. Kiessling KH, Piehl K, Lundquist CG: Number and size of skeletal muscle mitochondria in trained sedentary men. In: Coronary Heart Disease and Physical Fitness, ed. Larsen OA, Malmborg RO. Copenhagen, Munksgaard, 1971

9. Cooksey JD, Reilly P, Brown S, et al: Exercise training and plasma catecholamines in patients with ischemic heart disease. Am J Cardiol 42:372–376, 1978

10. Haskell WL: Mechanisms by which physical activity may enhance the clinical status of cardiac patients. pp. 276–296. In: Heart Disease and Rehabilitation, ed. Pollack ML, Schmidt DH. Boston, Houghton Mifflin, 1979

11. Rechnitzer PA, Yuhasz MS, Paivio A, et al: Effects of a 24-week exercise program on normal adults and patients with previous myocardial infarction. B Med J 1:734, 1967

12. Clausen JP, Klausen K, Rasmussen B, et al: Central and peripheral circulatory changes after training of the arms or legs. Am J Physiol 225:675–682, 1973

13. Badeer H: The genesis of cardiomegaly in strenuous athletic training: a new look. J Sports Med Phys Fitness 15:57–67, 1975

14. Pandolf KB, Burse RL, Goldman RF: Role of physical fitness in heat acclimatisation, decay and reinduction. Ergonomics, 20:399–408, 1977

15. Pyörälä K, Kävävä R, Punsar S, et al: A controlled study of the effects of 18 months' physical training in sedentary middle-aged men with high indexes of risk relative to coronary heart disease. In: Coronary Heart Disease and Physical Fitness, ed. Larsen Oa, Malmborg RO. Copenhagen, Munksgaard, 1971

16. Rosing DR, Brakman P, Redwood DR, et al: Blood fibrinolytic activity in man. Circ Res 27:171–184, 1970

17. Holloszy JO, Skinner JS, Toro G, Cureton TK: Effects of a six month program of endurance exercise of the serum lipids of middle-aged men. Am J Cardiol 14:753, 1964

18. Johnson RH, Walton JL, Krebs HA, Williamson DH: Metabolic fuels during and after severe exercise in athletes and nonathletes. Lancet 2:452, 1969

19. Erklens DW, Albers JJ, Hazzard WR, et al: Moderate exercise high density lipoprotein cholesterol in myocardial infarction survivors. Clin Res 26:158A, 1978

20. Forrester JS, Diamond GA, Swan HJC: Correlation classification of clinical and hemodynamic function after acute myocardial infarction. Am J Cardiol 39:137–145, 1977

21. Wallace AG, Rerych SK, Jones RH, et al: Effects of exercise training on ventricular function in coronary disease. Circulation, 58(Suppl II):197 1978

22. Thoren P: Left ventricular receptor activated by severe asphyxia and by coronary artery occlusion. Acta Physiol Scand 85:455–463, 1972

23. Hoskins TA, Habasevich RA: Cardiac rehabilitation: an overview. Phys Ther 58:1183–1190, 1978

24. Varnauskas E, Bergman H, Houk P, Björntorp P: Haemodynamic effects of physical training in coronary patients. Lancet 2:8, 1966
25. Clausen JP, Larsen OA, Trap-Jensen J: Physical training in the management of coronary artery disease. Circulation 40:143, 1969
26. Holmberg S: The influence of exercise and of pacing-induced tachycardia on coronary blood flow and myocardial oxygen consumption. pp. 489–499. In: Myocardial Blood Flow in Man, ed. Maseri A, Torino, Minerva Medica, 1972
27. Kiamura K, Jorgensen CR, Gobel FL, et al: Hemodynamic correlates of myocardial oxygen consumption during upright exercise. J Appl Physiol 32:516–522, 1972
28. Ferguson RJ, Petitclerc R, Choquette G, et al: Effect of physical training on treadmill exercise capacity, collateral circulation and progression of coronary disease. Am J Cardiol 34:764–769, 1974
29. Kennedy CC, Spiekerman RE, Lindsay MI, et al: One-year graduated exercise program for men with angina pectoris. Mayo Clin Proc 51:231–236, 1976
30. Selvester R, Camp J, Sanmarco M: Effects of exercise training on progression of documented coronary atherosclerosis in men. In: The Marathon; Physiological, Medical, Epidemiological, and Psychological Studies, ed. Milvy P. Ann NY Acad Sci 301:495–508, 1977
31. Egeberg O: The effect of exercise on the blood clotting system. Scand J Clin Lab Invest 15:8–15, 1963
32. Bassler T: Marathon running and immunity to atherosclerosis. In: The Marathon: Physiological, Medical, Epidemiological, and Psychological Studies, ed. Milvy P. Ann NY Acad Sci 301:579–592, 1977
33. Ferguson RJ, Cote P, Gauthier P, et al: Changes in exercise coronary sinus blood flow with training in patients with angina pectoris. Circulation 58:41–47, 1978
34. Holmgren A, Mossfeld F, Sjöstrand T, et al: Effect of training on work capacity, total hemoglobin, blood volume, heart volume, and pulse rate in recumbent and upright positions. Acta Med Scand 50:72–74, 1970
35. Roskamm H: Central circulatory adjustment to exercise in well-trained subjects. pp. 17–20. In: Coronary Heart Disease and Physical Fitness, ed. Larsen OA, Malmborg O. Copenhagen, Munksgaard, 1971
36. Folkow B: Role of sympathetic nervous system. In: Coronary Heart Disease and Physical Fitness, ed. Larsen OA, Malmborg RO. Copenhagen, Munksgaard, 1971
37. Clausen JP: Circulatory adjustments to dynamic exercise and effect of physical training in normal subjects and in patients with coronary disease. Prog Cardiovasc Dis 18:445–458, 1976
38. Detry JRM, Rousseau M, Vandenbroucke G, et al: Increased arteriovenous oxygen difference after physical training in coronary heart disease. Circulation 44:109–118, 1971
39. Blackburn H, Taylor HL, Hamrell B, et al: premature ventricular complexes induced by stress testing: their frequency and response to physical conditioning. Am J Cardiol 31:441–449, 1973
40. Hellerstein HK, Hornsten TR: Assessing and preparing the patient for return to a meaningful and productive life. J Rehabil 32:48, 1966
41. Shephard RJ: Cardiac rehabilitation in prospect. pp. 521–550. In: Heart Disease and Rehabilitation, ed. Pollock ML, Schmidt DH. Boston, Houghton Mifflin, 1979
42. Naughton J, Bruhn JG, Lategola MT: Effects of physical training on physiologic and behavioral characteristics of cardiac patients. Arch Phys Med Rehabil 49:131, 1968

4 | Chart Review and Physical Assessment Prior to Exercise

Marion B. Schoneberger
Bill Schoneberger
Brenda Rae Lunsford

In using an interdisciplinary approach to care of the patient with coronary artery disease, the physical therapist needs to have as much background information as possible. The patients medical chart is a primary source of this information; much can be gleaned from the physician and allied health team reports as well as from laboratory results. Other information is obtained through the physical therapy patient interview and physical assessment.

The objective of this chapter is to provide an overview of information to be obtained from the medical chart and physical therapy assessment of the patient with coronary artery disease. The primary areas covered include physiological impairment, risk factors, symptoms, and psychosocial factors.

CHART REVIEW

The physician's history and physical provides pertinent information concerning diagnosis, present symptoms, problems, and physical findings. Key information in the physician's history includes the onset and character of symptoms associated with cardiovascular disease. Common cardiovascular symptoms include chest discomfort or pain, dyspnea, orthopnea, paroxysmal nocturnal dyspnea, syncope, vertigo, fatigue, palpitations, edema, ascites, and intermittent claudication. In addition to noting the presence of any of these symptoms, it is important to note the description of each symptom, to aid in defining whether it is of cardiac origin or not. A risk factor profile and a history of prior illnesses or diseases related to the cardiovascular system are important to review, in addition to the physician's statements or comments concerning initial impression of the patient and his disease.

The physician's physical exam is reviewed for pertinent physical findings. The cardiovascular examination includes assessment of such items as color, edema, dyspnea, heart and lung sounds, neck veins, and arterial pulses.

The physician's progress notes also supply important information about the patient's hospitalization. Information important to the physical therapist includes reason for admission, a statement of diagnosis, and occurrence of significant events during the hospitalization. Post-myocardial infarction patients are classified as complicated or uncomplicated, based on the presence or absence of specific diagnostic findings within the first 4 days of admission, including:

1. continued cardiac ischemia or extension of myocardial infarction (MI).
2. disturbances of cardiac rhythm or conduction including ventricular tachycardia or fibrillation, persistent complex premature ventricular contractions, second or third degree atrioventricular (AV) block, rapid atrial arrhythmias, or persistent sinus tachycardia.
3. circulatory impairment including persistent hypotension, signs of cardiogenic shock, or right heart failure.
4. persistent left ventricular failure and pulmonary edema.

Knowledge of any of the above complications is critical for the physical therapy evaluation and treatment program. Patients who are still complicated by the end of the first 4 days have an increased risk of developing late serious hospital complications and death.[1]

Medications

Medications commonly prescribed for cardiac disease can be divided into five groups: cardiotonics, vasodilators, anti-hypertensives, anti-arrhythmics, and beta-blockers. The most common medications are:

1. digitalis—a cardiotonic given to treat congestive heart failure and for treatment of atrial arrhythmias.
2. nitroglycerin—a vasodilator taken sublingually during an episode of angina pectoris; it may also be prescribed to reduce diastolic pressure and therefore reduce the workload on the heart.
3. quinidine—the primary anti-arrhythmic prescribed to prevent both atrial and ventricular arrhythmias by prolonging the refractory period of the cardiac muscle cell.
4. propranolol—a beta-blocker which is used in the treatment of angina

pectoris, hypertension, and ventricular arrhythmias, and is effective because it blocks sympathetic nervous system of the heart.

5. hydrochlorothiazide—a diuretic that blocks the reabsorption of sodium and chloride ions in the kidney. It is prescribed for the treatment of hypertension and fluid retention.

Since all of these medications may affect the patient's ability to exercise, the physical therapist must be aware of the medications the patient is taking.

Various diagnostic studies and laboratory reports are found in the chart and provide useful information for the physical therapist. It is not necessary for the physical therapist to be able to interpret sophisticated diagnostic tests, but it is important to review the results or summary of the studies and understand how the information they can provide will influence the therapist's management of the patient.

Electrocardiogram

The electrocardiogram (ECG) is a recording of the electrical activity of the heart and is used to determine cardiac rhythm and conduction, diagnosis of specific chamber enlargement, and detection of myocardial ischemia or infarction. In addition, an estimate of the size or extent and location of the infarction is very desirable.

Vectorcardiogram

The vectorcardiogram is a multi-lead high gain three-dimensional ECG that provides a graphic display of the amplitude and direction of conduction through the myocardium. Accurate mapping of ventricular and septal conduction is also possible and is a more sophisticated technique for determining size and location of infarction.

Chest X-ray

The routine chest X-ray includes both frontal and left lateral projections and provides information regarding the cardiac silhouette, overall cardiac size, the cardiac thoracic ratio, and enlargement of specific chambers or the great vessels. Examination of the lung fields may reveal abnormalities of the lung parenchyma, infiltrates, emboli, congestion and/or evidence for increased left ventricular filling pressure, or fluid accumulation.

Ambulatory ECG

An ambulatory ECG is a two-lead 10 to 24 hour ECG recording. The patient wears a small magnetic tape recorder attached to the surface electrodes and keeps a diary of all activities during the time of the monitor. The tape is then scanned for ECG abnormalities, such as ST segment changes and/or complex arrhythmias, which are correlated with the specific activities occurring at the time of the abnormality.

Echocardiogram

An echocardiogram is a non-invasive procedure used to identify cardiac structures and the recording of their dynamic movements as a function of time. Ultrasound waves are transmitted from a transducer placed on the chest wall and reflected by underlying structures back to the transducer. The reflected impulses are displayed on an oscilloscope and recorded on paper. Echocardiography is particularly useful in the diagnosis of valvular heart disease but may also reflect abnormalities in chamber size and regional wall movement.[2]

Laboratory Reports

Enzyme studies are used to confirm the diagnosis of myocardial infarction. If the patient has had an infarct the enzyme report will show a rise in creatinephosphokinase (CPK) within 3 to 5 hours after the onset of chest pain and will peak by 30 hours. Serum glutamic oxaloacetic transaminase (SGOT) and lactate dehydrogenase (LDH) reach their peaks by the third and fourth days respectively. LDH is the slowest to return to baseline and may be elevated up to 8 to 12 days.

Additional laboratory studies provide useful information concerning total cholesterol and triglycerides, as well as lipoprotein fractionation and the ratio of total cholesterol to high density lipoprotein.

Radionuclide Studies

Radionuclides are used to determine the presence of acute myocardial ischemia, myocardial blood flow, and ventricular wall motion and function. After intravenous injection, one type of circulating radioisotope is taken up by viable myocardial cells while other types continue to circulate. The radioisotopes emit gamma photons which are detected by a nuclear instrument and recorded to provide a visual image of myocardial blood distribution or ventricular wall motion. The studies may be performed at rest to detect the early presence of infarction, or in combination with an exercise test to evaluate myocardial blood flow, segmental wall motion, and ejection fraction.[2]

Exercise Test

An exercise test is a standardized procedure used to define a patient's functional capacity and disclose the physiologic and symptomatic mechanisms that limit it. Results of the exercise test, either maximal or low level, should be carefully reviewed by the physical therapist and the following information obtained:

1. heart rate range
2. blood pressure range

3. type and frequency of arrhythmias
4. pre and post exercise heart sounds
5. ECG changes, including onset, duration, and degree of ST segment change
6. reason for stopping
7. time or workload completed
8. physical work capacity
9. symptoms

Cardiac Catheterization

A cardiac catheterization, when available, provides information about the anatomy and physiology of the heart. Selective cineangiocardiography involves the placement of a catheter into each coronary artery and injection of a radio-opaque dye. The arteriogram is a recording on cine film of the coronary artery anatomy, circulation, and the location and degree of obstruction in the arteries. The catheter then may be passed through the aortic valve into the left ventricle for the injection of dye. The ventriculogram is a recording of left ventricular wall motion and identifies areas of abnormal motion and the size and location of infarction.

A cardiac catheterization also provides additional information about intra-cardiac pressures and volumes of the ventricles, and ejection fraction. This information helps assess left ventricular function, which is critical to cardiac output and the activity tolerance of the patient (Figs. 4-1a, b, c).

Supplemental Chart Data

The physical therapist will find it necessary to review other allied health team members' reports (nursing, occupational therapy, social work, psychology) for their assessment and impression of the patient. Of special importance are patient responses to such self-care activities as bathing, grooming, and hygiene, as well as a thorough psychosocial profile. At the conclusion of the chart review the therapist should have a good understanding of the patient's medical and social history and be alert to special considerations in planning for the physical therapy evaluation of each patient.

PHYSICAL THERAPY ASSESSMENT

Following the chart review, each patient is thoroughly evaluated to plan a treatment program to meet his individual needs. A complete physical therapy evaluation includes an interview, physical examination, chest wall examination, and functional assessment.

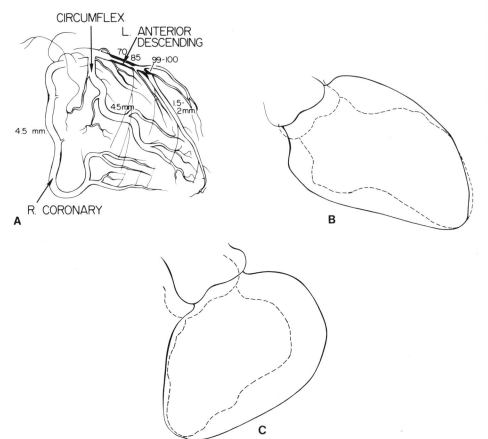

Fig. 4-1. (A) Selective coronary arteriography revealing 70–85 percent obstruction of the left anterior descending artery proximally and total occlusion distally. No significant lesions are seen in the circumflex or right coronary arteries. Artery diameters, important to the surgeon when considering bypass, are indicated in millimeters. (B) Ventriculogram, anterior oblique view. The solid line outlines the left ventricle at the end of diastole, the dotted line at the end of systole. (C) Ventriculogram, left lateral view. Viewed in combination (B and C), the ventriculogram reveals a large superior, anterior and apical akinetic segment consistent with a myocardial infarction secondary to total occlusion of the left anterior descending artery (A).

Interview

To add to the information obtained from the physician's clinical history and physical, it is necessary for the physical therapist to interview the patient. Special attention is given to prior life style and activity level, vocational and recreational interests, risk factor profile, knowledge of heart disease, assessment of pain, and personal goals.

The interview also plays an important part in establishing the patient-therapist relationship, which may be a key factor in compliance to the rehabilitation program. Observations of expressions and mannerisms as well as recognition of psychological and emotional overtones during the interview help the therapist learn more about the patient's acceptance and adaptation to his disease.[3]

During the interview the physical therapist identifies the patient's daily routine, including type and number of hours of work per week as well as attitude toward the job. Also discussed are leisure-time interests and activities. The patient is asked to identify the major problems or limitations interfering with his daily routine. In addition, a complete risk factor profile is obtained to supplement the chart review. This includes family history of coronary artery disease and diabetes, and personal history of hypertension, smoking, hyperlipidemia, obesity, stress, and sedentary life style.

This information provides the therapist with a clear picture of the patient's present functional level, previous life style, and what changes and modifications may be made. It is not uncommon to find a patient who needs to make several major modifications in his life style.

Discovering how much the patient understands about his disease is important so that appropriate education can be included in the treatment program. An understanding of the disease may be an important factor in both the anxiety level of the patient and compliance with the treatment program.

Questioning the patient about personal goals and expectations of himself and the treatment program allows the therapist to help the patient establish short and long-term goals concerning vocation and recreation that are realistically attainable.

It is important to assess carefully the history, location, and description of chest discomfort or pain. Specific questions about precipitating factors, frequency and duration of the discomfort, and relieving factors will help the therapist differentiate angina caused by myocardial ischemia from chest wall pain of a musculoskeletal origin, and assess the degree of limitation or interference with daily activities.

Getting a patient to describe angina is often difficult because the location may be vague; however, it usually is in the chest, neck, or arms, and is often described by the patient as a pressure, tightness, heaviness, or squeezing sensation rather than a pain. Angina is typically precipitated by or associated with eating, exercise, or emotional stress, and usually is relieved quickly when the cause is removed or a nitroglycerin is taken. It is also important to determine if angina is occurring more frequently, or being produced by less effort or even at rest or during sleep. This may be a sign of impending infarction.

In contrast to angina, chest wall pain is usually described as more distinctly located in a specific area, and is characteristically reported as a sharp knife-like or burning sensation, sensitive to palpation or deep breathing, and not specifically related to any such precipitating factors as eating, exercise, or emotional stress. The patient may report the pain lasting from a few minutes to as long as a few days.

Physical Examination

The physical examination includes an evaluation of strength, range of motion, and sensation of the trunk and extremities to make sure the patient has no extremity problems that may interfere with further testing or treatment. Balance, coordination, and gait are also important to evaluate since problems in these areas may interfere with exercise testing or treatment activities.

Chest Wall Examination

A chest wall inspection is performed with any patient who has a complaint of chest pain or discomfort. The purpose is to identify specific trigger areas of pain on the chest wall in order to distinguish chest wall pain from angina.

The examination is performed with fingerpoint palpation of the intercostal spaces 1 through 7, parasternal to the midclavicular line, along the infraclavicular space, and along the sternocleidomastoid and trapezius for tenderness which may be referring pain (Fig. 4-2). The examination also includes comparison of the patient's response to other less tender areas and the effects of maximum inspiration and expiration on the pain.

Functional Assessment

Following the interview and chest wall examination, an objective measurement of the patient's physiological response to the activities of daily living must be made. Several non-invasive measures can provide the physical therapist with

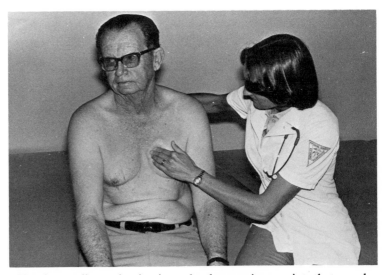

Fig. 4-2. The chest wall examination is used to locate trigger points that may be sensitive to palpation.

valuable information about how the damaged, ischemic, or revascularized myocardium is able to respond to the demands placed on it by increasing amounts of activity. These measures include: heart rate (pulse), blood pressure, abnormal rhythms or ST segment change on ECG, and chest auscultation for murmurs, changes in S_3, S_4 heart sounds, and/or pulmonary rales. Combined with clinical observation of signs and symptoms, these measures comprise the "clinical monitoring tools" that are necessary to perform routine physiological functional assessment.

Heart Rate. Heart rate (beats per minute), the easiest parameter to measure, is probably the best single indicator of the work being performed by the heart. Cardiac output (the volume of blood being pumped by the heart per minute) must increase as activity levels increase: walking or dressing require more cardiac output than sitting quietly. The heart is capable of increasing its output by increasing its rate of contraction and its stroke volume (the volume of blood pumped each beat). This is represented by the equation:

$$\text{Cardiac Output} = \text{Heart Rate} \times \text{Stroke Volume} \qquad (1)$$

Heart rate is most accurately determined measuring an ECG tracing, but when this is not available, the peripheral pulse is adequate. Pulse taken for 10 seconds and multiplied by 6 will be accurate to within 6 to 12 beats per minute. The radial pulse is the most common site, but the brachial and carotid pulses are often used. One must never apply bilateral pressure to the carotid pulses because of the potential compromise to cerebral blood flow (Fig. 4-3). An additional consideration when taking a pulse is its rhythm or regularity. Rhythm is normally regular at rest. Mild normal variation due to respiration (slowing with inspiration) is typically not perceptible to palpation. Any skips or pauses may indicate the presence

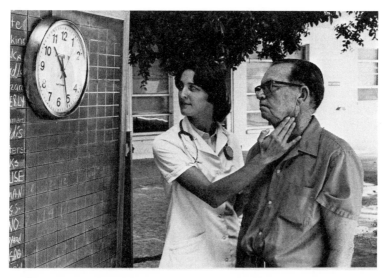

Fig. 4-3. When palpating the carotid pulse it is important to apply pressure to only one side of the neck.

of arrhythmias. To assess rhythm, pulse must be palpated for 1 to 2 minutes continuously to make any conclusive observations about the presence of arrhythmias. A good time to assess rhythm is immediately following an activity. Since one can detect only rhythm irregularity by palpation, however, and cannot be any more specific, it is imperative to monitor such patients with ECG to define the specific rhythm abnormality.

Blood Pressure.   The combination of heart rate and systolic blood pressure is the best non-invasive representation of work performed by the myocardium. The ability of the left ventricle to generate systolic pressure to deliver blood to the brain and the exercising muscle is a key factor in determining the pace and intensity of the rehabilitative process. Diastolic blood pressure represents the peripheral vascular system's ability to relax smooth muscle (vasodilate) and allow blood to flow where it is needed; therefore it usually does not rise or may even fall slightly during lower extremity activity.

The use of a mercury column sphygmomanometer with a long hose between the cuff and mercury column is recommended when a patient is exercising in a stationary position (egometer or treadmill). An anaeroid type is used for activities requiring mobility. An adult-sized cuff will usually suffice, but a thigh cuff may be needed with an obese patient.[4]

Because systolic blood pressure will begin dropping toward resting levels as soon as activity is stopped, it is important to obtain blood pressure readings within 15 to 20 seconds of terminating the activity. A technique that has proven useful when taking blood pressure on an ambulating subject is to ask the patient to walk in place while the reading is taken to prevent blood pooling in the lower extremities (Fig. 4-4). This will result in a more accurate reading. If the diaphragm of the stethoscope is placed over the area on the antecubital fossa where the brachial pulse is best felt, sounds are usually accentuated.

Electrocardiography.   While the heart rate and blood pressure provide primarily hemodynamic information, the elctrocardiogram supplies the clinician with electrophysiological insights. Radiotelemetry and/or direct hard wired ECG allow the observer to determine heart rate, rhythm, conduction, and repolarization patterns. Its most important use probably lies in the detection of dangerous arrhythmias and ischemic changes that may occur during activity or immediately following activity.

The use of ECG during functional assessment always requires two persons, often the therapist plus an assistant or aide. Both therapist and assistant must be able to recognize rapidly both normal ECG and its variations and abnormalities. The therapist remains with the patient to take blood pressure, assess symptoms, auscultate the chest before and after activity: the assistant remains with the ECG equipment to record periodic tracings, continually observe the oscilloscope, report heart rates to the therapist, and record blood pressures. Ten to 15-second ECG tracings are recorded pre- and post-exercise, at regular intervals during the functional assessment (every 1, 3, and 5 minutes), with each new activity (lower extremity dressing, ambulation), and whenever significant arrhythmias, conduction disturbances, or ischemic changes are observed on the oscilloscope. For the latter

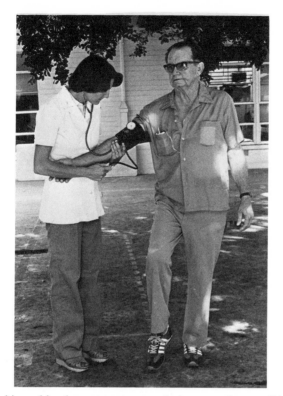

Fig. 4-4. When taking a blood pressure on an ambulatory patient, walking in place while the reading is taken prevents blood pooling in the legs that could cause a low reading.

reason, a telemetered system with a short (6-10 seconds) memory capability is preferred so that any abnormality observed on the oscilloscope can be recorded for documentation, closer inspection, and review by the therapist and/or physician. The individual responsible for recording heart rate, blood pressure, symptoms, type of activity, and time elapsed can do so directly on the ECG paper so that all of the physiological findings can be correlated when these objective findings are reviewed at a later time.

Chest Auscultation.   Information regarding heart and lung sounds can be found in the physician's physical report, but the physical therapist should also be capable of identifying normal and some abnormal chest sounds. This skill is especially useful during the initial evaluation and early weeks of rehabilitation, when complications are most likely to occur and auscultatory findings may be the first objective evidence.

Equipment and techniques.   The stethoscope with a short tube (10 to 12 inches) connected to each ear piece and equipped with both a diaphragm and a bell is preferred. The single tube stethoscope is preferred especially for taking blood pressures on exercising subjects. The diaphragm is used to accentuate high

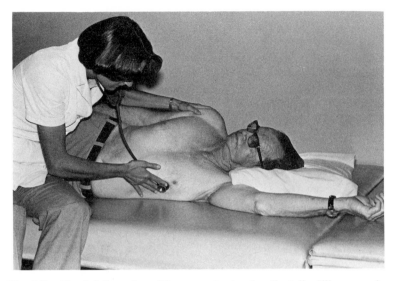

Fig. 4-5. The left lateral position accentuates the diastolic filling sounds.

frequency sounds and when used should be pressed tightly against the skin. The bell will accentuate low frequency sounds, but light pressure, only enough to make a seal with the skin, should be used.

Although the human ear is capable of hearing sounds from 20 to 20,000 Hz, it is most sensitive to sounds in the 1,000 to 5,000 Hz range. Most clinical cardiovascular sounds are in the range below 1,000 Hz. Because of this natural disadvantage, every attempt must be made to accentuate the heart sounds. The patient should be examined in a quiet room with all areas of the chest easily accessible to the stethoscope. Because in the sitting or standing position blood can pool in the lower extremities, initial auscultation should be performed with the patient in the supine position, and in specific cases in the left lateral position where some sounds are best heard (Fig. 4-5).

Heart sounds are best identified if a system for auscultation is used. The following system is recommended:

1. Start at the apex of the heart (4th or 5th intercostal space in the mid-clavicular line) and slowly move the diaphragm to the left sternal border in a stepwise fashion, then cephalad to the base of the heart. Listen in the pulmonic area (second left intercostal space) and the aortic area (second right intercostal space).

2. Identify the first heart sound and determine if splitting is occurring.

3. Identify the second heart sound and try to identify the separate aortic (A_2) and pulmonic (P_2) closure components.

4. Listen for extra sounds first during systole and then during diastole using both diaphragm and bell.

5. Auscultate the posterior chest for breath sounds in the sitting position.

The first heart sound. Caused by closure of the mitral and tricuspid valves, the first heart sound (S_1) is best heart at the apex with the diaphragm. The first heart sound signals the beginning of systole. A normal (physiological) splitting of the first sound may be heard because the left ventricle may contact slightly before the right, and therefore the mitral valve will close before the tricuspid.

The second heart sound. Caused by closure of the aortic and pulmonic valves, the second heart sound (S_2) is best heard at the base of the heart. S_2 signals the end of systole and the beginning of diastole. At slow heart rates, systole is shorter than diastole; therefore differentiation of the first from the second heart sound becomes possible. Because the systolic ejection time in the right ventricle is longer than the left, the pulmonic closure sound (P_2) is heard after the aortic closure sound (A_2). This splitting, best heard in the pulmonic area, is also physiologic and will be widened during inspiration (Fig. 4-6a). Wider than normal splitting of S_2 will be heard with right bundle branch block. The S_2 may be paradoxically split (P_2 precedes A_2) with left bundle branch block, aortic stenosis, and patent ductus arteriosus. In this case, however, the wider splitting will occur during expiration (Fig. 4-6b).

Diastolic filling sounds (gallop rhythms). During the initial opening of the atrioventricular valves, called early passive rapid filling, a third heart sound (S_3) can sometimes be heard in children and young adults and is normal. It is probably caused by vibration of the valve leaflets and chordae tendineae. A pathological S_3 can be heard in the older adult and may signal ventricular failure or valve incompetence. This may be one of the only external signs of myocardial dysfunction and is caused by the rapid flow of blood into a dilated non-compliant ventricle. It is best heard at the apex, using the bell, with the patient in the left lateral position. It is heard following the second heart sound in early to mild diastole and therefore causes the heart to sound like a galloping horse (Fig. 4-6c). An S_3 is most significant if heard after activity.

A fourth heart sound (S_4) is often heard in patients with hypertension, coronary artery disease, cardiomyopathy, and aortic stenosis. It occurs in late diastole during the late rapid active filling phase and is caused by atrial contraction (systole) into a non-compliant ventricle. It is commonly heard in patients with post-myocardial infarction.[5] It too is best heard with the patient in the left lateral position, using the bell over the left sternal border or the apex.

At times both an S_3 and S_4 will be present and may blend together with rapid heart rates into what has been called a summation gallop, making it difficult to identify specifically any of the heart sounds.

Murmurs. A detailed discussion of murmurs is beyond the scope of this book, but in general they are caused by a turbulent flow of blood through normal or abnormal valves. It may be forward flow through a constricted or irregular valve, or backward regurgitant flow through an incompetent valve, septal defect, or patent ductus arteriosus. Murmurs are classified according to timing (systolic/diastolic), intensity (grades I to VI), location (apex, base, axilla), and radiation (e.g. apex to axilla).

To the clinician involved in cardiac rehabilitation, the two most significant

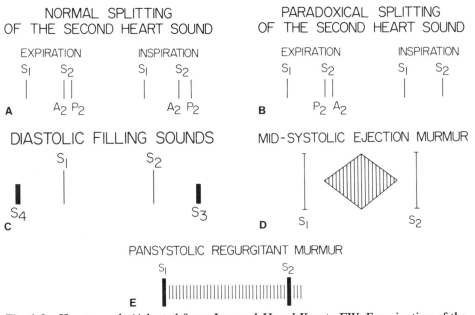

Fig. 4-6.   Heart sounds.(Adapted from: Leonard JJ and Kroety FW: Examination of the Heart: Auscultation. American Heart Association, 1974)

murmurs both occur during systole. The first is the systolic ejection murmur of aortic stenosis. It is heard best in the second right and second and third left intercostal spaces, and radiates to the neck and carotid arteries. Its intensity builds to a peak at mid-systole and then decreases and stops prior to S_2 (Fig. 4-6d). A grade III or greater systolic ejection murmur may be hemodynamically significant, representing a potential reduction in cardiac output. Patients with severe aortic stenosis are prone to syncopal attacks and even sudden death.

The second murmur is the pansystolic murmur of mitral valve insufficiency. Heard best at the apex, it is a soft, blowing sound that radiates to the axilla. It does not build in intensity (Fig. 4-6e). When loud, it may replace the first heart sound and may continue up to and through A_2, because even after aortic valve closure, left ventricular pressure may exceed left atrial pressure, allowing regurgitant flow to continue. Mitral valve insufficiency may be found in patients following myocardial infarction that has caused papillary muscle damage and/or rupture of the chordae tendineae. These patients may be prone to left heart failure; therefore an increase in intensity of this murmur may be of clinical significance.

Breath sounds.   The physical therapist should be able to differentiate normal inspiratory and expiratory breath sounds with the diaphragm placed on the patient's back from the area of T1 through T10. Probably the only adventitious (abnormal) breath sounds of clinical significance in cardiac rehabilitation are rales. These are sometimes present with pulmonary edema secondary to left heart failure. Often heard best at the bases of the lungs, these are crackling sounds heard during inspiration, caused by partially fluid filled alveoli popping open.

Physical therapists new to chest auscultation will need to enlist the aid of physicians when learning this skill. It is best to verify the presence of an extra heart or lung sound. As with most skills, accuracy improves with experience.

Signs and Symptoms. In addition to the specific monitoring just described, listening to patient complaints, observing the patient carefully, and periodic questioning are important components of a thorough ongoing evaluation process. There are four major areas of concern:

1. myocardial infarction, which may be signaled by angina pectoris (discussed previously).

2. cardiac insufficiency and/or congestive heart failure. Onset or worsening may be indicated by a significant increase in S_4 or S_3 heart sounds with moderate activity such as walking and by symptoms such as shortness of breath with exertion and generalized fatigue. Orthopnea, which requires the subject to sleep with the head and thorax elevated, and distended neck veins develop as late signs in the disease. If the congestive heart failure is right-sided or if left-sided congestive heart failure becomes severe enough, the patient may develop ascites or pitting edema in the lower extremities as fluid backs up in the venous system.

3. arrhythmias, which may be identified by patients reporting a feeling of palpitations, episodes of vertigo, or even syncopal attacks. A long burst of ventricular tachycardia or even frequent premature ventricular contractions may result in reduced cardiac output and poor perfusion to the brain. Immediate ECG monitoring is indicated when patients complain of these symptoms.

4. peripheral vascular disease, often picked up when the patient complains of a cramping, burning pain in the calves or buttocks during activity (walking) that is relieved with rest. The discomfort of muscle fatigue secondary to deconditioning will be relieved as the days pass, but intermittent claudication will continue to occur or become worse as the activity becomes more strenuous.

These "clinical monitoring tools," used in combination, provide valuable information to the physical therapist, the physician, and the patient about the ability of the compromised heart and cardiovascular system to adapt safely to the demands of functional activities. When such activities (i.e., self-care activities, walking, stair climbing, yard work) are done in a standardized way, they provide reproducible, objective evidence of both candidacy for and progression through a cardiac rehabilitation program.

ASSESSMENT SUMMARY

The goal of the assessment is to bring together all the information from the chart review, interview, and evaluation to determine the patient's major problems (Fig. 4-7). Assessment of four major problem areas is critical to being able to correctly determine goals and develop a treatment plan.

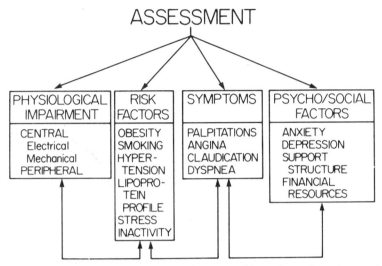

Fig. 4-7. Assessment involves the identification of problems from these four major areas and the determination of their effect on the treatment program.

Physiological Impairment

Physiological impairment that will affect the patient's ability to exercise may be related to either central or peripheral sources, or both. Central sources of impairment may be strictly mechanical or may be electrical problems that have mechanical effects.

Since the heart's job is simply to provide adequate cardiac output for the peripheral needs, any pathological problem that impairs cardiac output will affect activity tolerance. Common mechanical problems are large or massive infarction, aortic stenosis, mitral insufficiency, systemic hypertension, persistent myocardial ischemia (especially with exercise), and cardiomyopathy. Information concerning central mechanical impairment is drawn from the various diagnostic tests (12-lead ECG, vectorcardiogram, echocardiogram, radionuclide studies, and cardiac catheterization), physical findings (presence of congestive heart failure), and, most importantly, from the functional assessments (physiological monitoring and stress testing). The heart's ability to provide blood to the periphery will be reflected by adequate heart rate and systolic blood pressure responses to activity, without signs of pump failure as the activity levels are increased. The primary electrical problems are arrhythmias. They may be potentially fatal, or if they occur frequently enough may also reduce cardiac output and exercise capacity. Information concerning electrical complications begins with coronary care unit monitoring and is supplemented by the functional monitoring that follows (ambulatory ECG, radiotelemetry ECG, and stress testing). Arrhythmias that may affect cardiac output include: any supraventricular or ventricular tachycardias, brachycardia, second and third degree AV block, atrial fibrillation/flutter with rapid ventricular rate, and frequent premature supraventricular and ventricular ectopics. Any arrhythmia that increases in frequency or is induced by exercise will potentially limit exercise tolerance and must be further evaluated.

Peripheral factors that will affect exercise capacity relate to the vascular system's ability to adapt to exercise and the ability of the exercising muscles to perform work. Problems related to peripheral maladaptation are: diastolic hypertension, systolic hypertension, intermittent claudication, and angina pectoris. All of these are best assessed during activity. Peripheral muscle deconditioning secondary to bed rest or inactive life style and occasional neurological orthopedic problems are the most common non-vascular causes for reduced exercise tolerance.

Risk Factors

Effective treatment of coronary disease involves modification of lifestyles that are known to exacerbate the disease process. One would expect major lifestyle changes to be more difficult than minor ones. The patient whose risk factor profile includes a long history of heavy smoking, obesity, hypertension, sedentary life style, and job-related stress may find the rehabilitation process more difficult than a patient who has only one risk factor, and may therefore require more specific goal setting on the physical therapist's part.

Symptoms

The major symptoms seen in patients with coronary artery disease are dyspnea, angina pectoris, fatigue, and claudication. Any patient who exhibits these symptoms any time in the assessment process must be considered more closely. The linking of symptoms with objective findings accentuates the importance of the functional assessment; for example, ST depression with angina. One of the more important criteria when considering elective coronary bypass surgery is the functional limitations imposed by angina pectoris. The physical therapist's assessment at the functional level can help provide the physician with this information.

Psychosocial Factors

The emotional implications of heart disease are well known. Anxiety and depression are the two most common psychological side effects seen in the patient after myocardial infarction.[6] The physical therapist who is aware that these side effects exist and is comfortable with the behavior changes that frequently accompany them will be able to provide more adequate patient care. The patient who has good family support and is not under financial strain will be more capable of making important lifestyle changes than the patient who is not as fortunate.

In summary, the assessment of rehabilitation potential requires the blending of information gleaned from the patient's clinical history, diagnostic tests, interview, and physiological monitoring of functional activity. Potential roadblocks to recovery include physiological impairment and symptoms secondary to the disease process, patient lifestyle that may cause further risk, and psychosocial complications secondary to or in addition to heart disease.

REFERENCES

1. McNeer JF, et al: The course of acute myocardial infarction; feasibility of early discharge of the uncomplicated patient. Circulation 51:410–413, 1975
2. Vanden Belt RJ, et al: Cardiology: A Clinical Approach. Year Book Medical Publishers, 1979
3. Silverman ME: Examination of the Heart: The Clinical History. American Heart Association, 1975
4. Geddes LA, Tiuey R: The importance of cuff width in measurement of blood pressure indirectly. Cardiovasc Res Cent Bull 14 (3): 69–79, Jan–March, 1976
5. Leonard JJ, Kroety FW: Examination of the Heart: Auscultation. American Heart Association, 1974
6. Cassem NH and Hackett TP: Psychological rehabilitation of myocardiac infarction patients in the acute phase. Heart Lung 2 (3), 382–388, 1973

5 | Electrocardiography

Marcia J. Pearl

THE CONDUCTION SYSTEM

SA Node and Atrial Pathways

The sinoatrial (SA) node is a specialized group of cells located 1 millimeter beneath the right atrial epicardium at its junction with the superior vena cava. It is 20 millimeters long and is elliptical in shape. The SA node has a resting membrane potential of 55 to 60 millivolts compared to the resting membrane potential of 75 to 90 millivolts found in other conducting tissues. The SA node is the pacemaker of the heart because a lower threshold potential necessitates less stimulus to evoke an action potential, and because the SA node recovers more rapidly, resulting in rapid rhythmicity.

Once the SA node has been stimulated, the wave of depolarization travels at .3 m/sec in all directions away from the stimulus. From the SA node, the cardiac impulse spreads rapidly throughout the right atrium and to the left ventricle along a special pathway called Bachmann's Bundle.[1] This specialized intraatrial myocardial band conducts impulses from the SA node to the left atrium. Impulses from the SA to the atrioventricular (AV) node are conducted along three tracts or internodal bundles: the anterior internodal tract or bundle of Kent, the middle internodal tract or Wenckebach bundle, and the posterior internodal tract or Thorel's bundle.[1] The depolarization of the atria is represented as the P wave on the ECG.

AV Node and Ventricular System

The AV node is situated beneath the endocardium of the right atrium above the septal leaflet of the tricuspid valve. The AV node includes the Bundle of His.

When the impulse reaches the AV node, conduction is slowed markedly. There is a .10 second pause before the impulse actually stimulates the AV node,

61

which allows blood to pass through the AV valves. This pause is represented as the isoelectric line on the ECG between the P wave and the beginning of the QRS complex and is known as the P-R interval.

After the pause, the AV node receives the depolarization stimulus from the atria. The AV node is stimulated and the stimulus proceeds through the AV node to the Bundle of His and to the Bundle Branches. The Bundle of His passes down the right side of the interventricular septum and then divides into the right and left bundle branches. The right bundle branch (RBB) is a direct continuation of the Bundle of His and proceeds down the right side of the interventricular septum. The left bundle branch (LBB) arises almost perpendicularly from the Bundle of His and perforates the interventricular septum on the subendocardial surface of the left side of the interventricular septum. The LBB is considerably thicker than the RBB. This thickened tissue splits into a thin anterior division and a thick posterior division. The Bundle Branches then merge into a profusely branching terminal network called the Purkinje fibers. The Purkinje fibers simultaneously depolarize both ventricles.

Blood Supply to the Conduction System

Blood supply to the SA node is via the SA node artery, a branch of the left circumflex in about 45 percent of the population, and a branch of the right coronary artery (RCA) in 55 percent of the population.[2] All but the smallest atrial infarctions are associated with occlusion of the flow to the SA node artery. Such occlusion also causes infarction of the sinus node and can lead to atrial arryhthmias. The occlusion is rarely in the SA node artery itself, but rather in the main coronary artery proximal to the origin of the SA node artery.

The AV node artery is supplied by the RCA in 90 percent of the population, and in 10 percent of the population by the circumflex.[2] The AV nodal artery supplies the AV node, Bundle of His, and proximal right and left bundle branches. The bundle branches are supplied by the septal arteries arising from the left anterior descending artery.

THE STANDARD ECG

Description

The ECG is usually recorded on ruled paper. This provides a means for measuring both the magnitude and duration of the heart's electrical events. The paper is ruled both horizontally and vertically in 1 mm lines. Each fifth line is thicker to allow a visual aid in measurement. The horizontal axis measures time and the vertical axis measures amplitude. The paper is calibrated so that one inch equals one second. Each inch in turn is broken into five segments by a dark vertical line; each segment is 1/5 of a second or .20 second. These fifths are further divided into five smaller segments representing .04 second. Thus 25 small squares equal one second. The paper speed of the ECG is generally 25 mm/sec and amplitude is measured on the vertical axis. Each horizontal line represents a voltage change of .1 mv. Ten lines equals 1 mv.

The standard ECG is composed of 12 leads: three standard limb leads designated I, II, III; three augmented limb leads designated AVR, AVL, AVF; and six vector leads designated V_1, V_2, V_3, V_4, V_5, V_6. The limb leads are referred to as the frontal plane leads.

By convention, in lead I the negative electrode is on the right arm and the positive electrode is on the left arm. In lead II, the negative electrode is on the right arm and the positive electrode on the left leg. In lead III, the negative electrode is on the left arm and the positive electrode on the left leg. Each lead is derived from two points which are referred to as bipolar electrodes.

In the augmented leads, the same electrode location is used as in the standard limb leads. However, the negative electrode is formed by combining leads I, II, and III to form an algebraic sum of zero. Therefore the leads measure the difference in potential between the limb and the center of the heart.

The ECG records the same activity in each lead. The waves appear different because the various leads monitor the activity from different vantage points.

The precordial leads record the activity of the heart as seen from the horizontal plane. These are unipolar leads with the negative pole projecting through the AV node towards the patient's back. Lead V_2 describes a straight line from the anterior to posterior of the patient.

By convention, V_1 is in the fourth intercostal space at the right sternal border; V_2 is in the fourth intercostal space at the left sternal border; V_3 is midway between V_2 and V_4; V_4 is in the fifth intercostal space at the mid-clavicular line; V_5 is in the fifth intercostal space at the anterior axillary line; and V_6 is in the fifth intercostal space at the mid-axillary line.

There are three basic laws of ECG that predict the wave formation:

1. A wave of depolarization spreading toward the positive electrode of any lead will inscribe a positive deflection. The more parallel the wave of excitation to the lead that inscribes it, the greater the deflection.

2. A wave of depolarization spreading toward the negative electrode of any lead will inscribe a negative deflection. The more parallel the wave of excitation to the lead that inscribes it, the greater the deflection.

3. A wave of depolarization that is perpendicular to any lead will inscribe a small diphasic deflection.

The deflections are named by convention, using the letters P, Q, R, S, T. An initial small rounded deflection is a P wave. It may be upright or inverted. A tall upright deflection is an R wave. A Q wave is any negative deflection preceding an R wave. It is not always present, but is the first wave of the complex when present. An S wave is any negative deflection following an R wave, or any downward stroke preceded by an upward stroke. Thus, the Q wave is a negative deflection preceding an R wave. The S wave is any negative deflection following an R wave. By convention a totally negative complex is called a QS complex.

The wave of ventricular depolarization is represented by the QRS complex. However, it is not necessary for all components of the wave to exist.

Normal Configuration

The P wave represents atrial depolarization. It is associated with normal transmission of an impulse originating in the SA node. It is normally upright in leads I, II, AVF and inverted in AVR. It should be gently rounded and 1 to 3 millivolts in amplitude. The duration of the normal P wave is .08 to .12 seconds.

The P-R interval is measured from the beginning of the P wave to the beginning of the QRS complex. It represents conduction just prior to the wave of depolarization leaving the Purkinje fibers. It is normally .12 to .20 seconds in duration; it may shorten with rapid heart rates. A P-R interval of greater duration indicates a conduction delay in the AV node.

The QRS complex represents ventricular depolarization. The Q wave represents the initial septal depolarization by the Bundle of His and bundle branches, and the RS represents the completion of ventricular activation by the Purkinje fibers. The normal duration of the QRS complex is .06 to .10 seconds. If the duration is increased it is a sign of delayed, abnormal conduction. The QRS complex can show a variable pattern in the extremity leads I, II, III, AVF, AVL. Lead AVR normally inscribes a negative QRS complex. In the precordial leads the R wave tends to become larger moving from V_1 to V_6, and the S wave becomes smaller. The maximum amplitude in the precordial leads should be 25 to 30 millivolts. Increased amplitude indicates ventricular hypertrophy. Amplitudes less than 5 millivolts may indicate coronary artery disease, emphysema, marked obesity, generalized edema, or pericardial effusion.

The ST segment describes the period between ventricular depolarization and ventricular repolarization. This corresponds to the refractory period of the action potential. Normally the segment is isoelectric but may be elevated 1 mm. It is never normally depressed greater than 1/2 mm. Severe elevation or depression indicate ischemia or infarction. Prolonged ST segment elevation may indicate a ventricular aneurysm. The ST segment normally curves gently and imperceptibly into the T wave. It should not be sharply angled, nor should it be frankly horizontal.

The T wave represents repolarization of the ventricle. As a rule it follows in the same direction as the QRS deflection. Its shape is slightly rounded; T waves which are sharply pointed or notched may indicate injury. The normal amplitude is less than 5 mm in the limb leads and less than 10 mm in the precordial leads. Extremely tall T waves are seen in patients with cerebral-vascular accidents and in myocardial infarctions.

As a general rule the P-QRS-T pattern in lead I resembles AVL; lead II resembles AVF. Lead II and AVR show reverse patterns.

INTERPRETING THE ECG

Determining the Rate

When reviewing a given ECG the first procedure that should be performed is to calculate the rate. This may be done by four methods:

1. Count the number of R waves in a 6 inch strip and multiply by 10. Since 6 inches equals 6 seconds, this is a reasonable method if the rhythm is regular.
2. Find an R wave that falls on a heavy black line. Count the number of large boxes (.20) between two successive R waves and divide that number into 300.
3. Find an R wave that falls on a vertical line. Count the number of small boxes between successive R waves and divide that number into 1500. Since there are 5 large boxes in 1 second, in 60 seconds there would be 300 large boxes. Since there are 25 small boxes in 1 second, in 60 seconds there would be 1500 small boxes.
4. Using the second method, one would find that if the successive R wave was one box away the rate would be 300, if two boxes away 150. The lines can be assigned numbers and memorized. Thus, if the successive R wave falls between two dark lines, the small boxes can be divided into the difference and given a value. Thus, $300 - 150 = 150$, and each small box equals 30. Example: the difference between 100 and 75 is 25; each small box is worth 5. Thus the rate would be 85 if an R wave fell on the second small line. Having calculated the ventricular rate, calculate the atrial rate and see if the ventricular and atrial rates are equal.

Rate and Rhythm Disturbances

By definition any rate greater than 100 is a tachycardia, and any rate slower than 60 is a bradycardia. Rate disturbances are not necessarily pathologic.

The pathophysiologic consequences of rate and rhythm disturbances are determined by:

1. the site of origin of cardiac impulse
2. length of diastolic filling time
3. atrial transport function
4. mechanical response
5. ability of the heart and peripheral circulation to compensate for alterations in cardiac output.

The normal resting subject will have little difficulty in circulatory homeostasis unless the heart rate drops below 40 or rises above 160. However, patients with pathology of the heart or blood vessels may not have the reserve to tolerate extremes of tachycardia or bradycardia because of decreased cardiac output, hypotension, and diminished blood flow.

Tachyarrhythmias have a double-barrel effect. Myocardial oxygen demand is directly proportional to heart rate. Thus, as the rate increases, demand for oxygen also increases, necessitating an increase in coronary blood flow. The coronary arteries obtain their blood supply during diastole; as heart rate increases, diastolic filling time decreases. If the coronary arteries are obstructed secondary to atherosclerosis, they may not have the ability to vasodilate, and the myocardial blood supply may be insufficient for the increased demand, causing myocardial ischemia.

Normal Sinus Rhythm (NSR)

Rate: 60–100

Rhythm: constant R-R interval

ECG Appearance: P-R interval .12 to .20 and constant. P wave is smooth, gently rounded, and symmetrical, 1 to 3 millivolts in amplitude. P wave is .08 to .12 seconds in duration. There is a P wave preceding each QRS. The P is upright in lead II, inverted in AVR. The QRS is of normal duration, .06 to .10, and of normal amplitude (Fig. 5-1).

Cause: the SA node is the origin of the impulses. It discharges regularly and conduction follows a normal pathway.

Signs and Symptoms: none

Clinical Significance: normal

Treatment: none

Sinus Tachycardia

Rate: 100–160

Rhythm: regular; constant R-R interval

ECG Appearance: as in NSR. The only difference is increased rate (Fig. 5-2).

Cause: normal origin of impulse from SA node but increased rate of discharge, primarily due to increased sympathetic nerve activity. Likely causes: fever, anxiety, apprehension, increased physical activity. Pathology: hypoxia, hemorrhage, hypotension, shock, infection, hyperthyroidism, heart failure, myo-

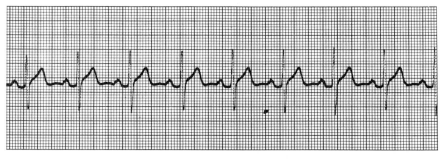

Fig. 5-1. Normal sinus rhythm.

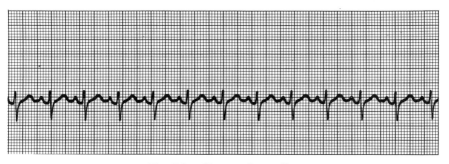

Fig. 5-2. Sinus tachycardia.

cardial infarction. Normal finding in infancy. Pharmacologic agents: atropine (decreases vagal tone), epinephrine, Isuprel (increases sympathetic tone), alcohol, nicotine, and caffeine.

Signs and Symptoms: none may be present if patient is able to compensate, or the patient may describe palpitations and dyspnea.

Clinical Significance: generally this arrhythmia is not significant. The increased heart rate does increase myocardial oxygen requirement and may promote angina or congestive heart failure in the compromised patient. The rapid rate may be potentially harmful in acute myocardial infarction since it decreases diastolic filling time.

Treatment: rest and treatment of the underlying causative factor(s).

Sinus Bradycardia

Rate: 40–60

Rhythm: regular; constant R-R interval

ECG Appearance: as in NSR. The only difference is diminished rate (Fig. 5-3).

Cause: may be a normal variant in well-trained individuals, during sleep, and with a valsalva phenomenon. Pathologic: increased vagal stimulus due to vomiting; hypothermia; meningitis and other sources of increased intracranial pressure such as tumor, hemorrhage, acute cerebral vascular accident, and glau-

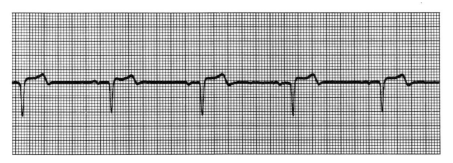
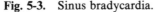

Fig. 5-3. Sinus bradycardia.

coma; jaundice; severe mental depression; inferior wall myocardial infarction; and hypothyroidism. Pharmacologic: can be caused by morphine, reserpine, Inderal, or Digoxin.

Signs and Symptoms: no symptoms present unless cardiac output cannot be sustained; then lightheadedness, dizziness, postural hypotension, and syncope may ensue.

Clinical Significance: a slow heart rate may allow an irritable ectopic focus to occur. The patient may not be able to maintain adequate cardiac output, particularly with exercise, and will complain of fatigue and lightheadedness. The skin may be cold and clammy as a result of shunting of blood from periphery to vital organs to maintain cardiac output.

Treatment: discontinue medications if they are probable cause. Give atropine to decrease vagal tone or Isuprel to increase sympathetic tone and enhance sinus node discharge. Treatment is necessary only if decreased heart rate is compromising the patient.

Arrhythmias Originating in the Atria

The atria, AV node, and ventricles all have the potential capacity to serve as pacemakers, but the SA node normally retains control, because its rate of recovery is faster than the other sites and its threshold is lower.

When the impulse originates in the atria, outside the SA node, at rates of 200 or less the P waves are visible but distorted, indicating that the SA node is not discharging. With rates up to 200, impulses reach and pass through the AV node without difficulty and a normal QRS follows.

With rates from 200 to 400, the AV node cannot accept every impulse and blocks every second or third beat. Those impulses that are transmitted through the AV node are conducted normally. When the atrial rate is greater than 400 times per minute, the AV node is no longer able to respond to each stimulus and impulses reach the AV node in an irregular fashion; therefore, the ventricular rhythm is irregular as well, although the QRS complex is normal in appearance.

It should be noted that blood normally flows continually from the great veins into the atria, and that ordinarily 70 percent of this venous return flows directly into the ventricles even before the atria contract. The atrial contraction causes an additional 30 percent filling known as the atrial kick. Therefore the primary function of the atria is to increase the effectiveness of the ventricle as a pump. Normally, loss of the atrial kick does not interfere with cardiac output; however, with exercise, loss of the atrial kick may markedly diminish cardiac output.

Premature Atrial Contractures (PAC)

Premature beats originate in an atrial ectopic focus, producing an abnormal P wave earlier than expected.

Rate: normal, but determined by basic rate and frequency of PACs.

Rhythm: normal except for the PAC which occurs earlier than anticipated. R-R is regular except for PACs.

ECG Appearance: because impulse does not originate in the SA node, the P wave is abnormally shaped or inverted, and differs from the normal contour of SA node origin P waves. Occasionally no clear P wave is seen. The QRS complex is of normal configuration and duration. Usually, the interval inscribed between the PAC and the next sinus P wave is only slightly longer than one P-P interval. This is a non-compensatory pause. The pause after the PAC is not long enough to make the interval between the two sinus initiated P waves flanking the PAC equal to twice the basic P-P interval.

Cause: may be normal; seen in emotional stress, excessive caffeine, nicotine, alcohol, and lack of sleep. Pathologic: arteriosclerotic disease, myocardial infarction, ischemia, hypertension, acute and chronic rheumatic fever, syphilitic heart disease, cardiac failure, and hyperthyroidism. Pharmacologic: may be caused by barium, calcium, epinephrine, digitalis toxicity.

Signs and Symptoms: usually none; patient may describe palpitations or skipped beats. Positive identification can be made only by ECG.

Clinical Significance: the arrhythmia is not significant, except that it represents atrial irritability which may forewarn of more serious arrhythmias, such as atrial fibrillation. More than six PACs per minute assumes greater importance. PACs may decrease cerebral blood flow as much as 8 percent, coronary flow by 5 percent, and renal flow 8 to 10 percent.[3]

Treatment: sedation; omit caffeine, alcohol, tobacco. Generally Digoxin, quinidine, or procainamide are used.

Paroxysmal Atrial Tachycardia (PAT)

Paroxysmal atrial tachycardia is a sudden rapid heart rate which usually arises from an ectopic pacemaker.

Rate: 150–250. Atrial and ventricular rates are identical.

Rhythm: regular; constant R-R interval

ECG Appearance: P wave may not be visible. It may be buried in the QRS complex or T wave, or if visible may not have a normal configuration. The P wave does not originate in the sinus node. The QRS configuration is normal since conduction beyond the AV node is normal (Fig. 5-4).

Cause: may be caused by caffeine, cigarettes, and alcohol. It is mediated by the autonomic nervous system as a manifestation of anxiety.

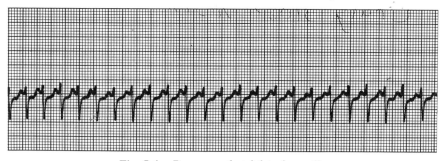

Fig. 5-4. Paroxysmal atrial tachycardia.

Signs and Symptoms: characteristically occurs suddenly and without warning. Patients describe a rapid fluttering, pounding sensation. PAT may be associated with dyspnea or tachypnea. The patient may complain of light-headedness. PAT ends as spontaneously as it starts.

Clinical Significance: none in the healthy patient. The rapid rate associated with PAT may be deleterious in ischemic heart disease. Increased heart rate may cause congestive heart failure in the poorly compensated patient. Hypotension and cardiogenic shock may ensue. The rhythm may decrease renal flow up to 18 percent and cerebral blood flow by as much as 23 percent.[3]

Treatment: carotid sinus massage or eyeball pressure for the oculo-cardiac reflex will stimulate the vagus nerve and return the patient to a normal sinus rhythm, although this effect may be transitory. Sedation, valsalva phenomenon, digitalis, propranolol, quinidine, procaine, cardioversion. The differential diagnosis of PAT is distinguished from all other atrial arrhythmias by its absolutely regular appearance and disappearance with carotid sinus stimulation.

Atrial Flutter

Atrial flutter is a tachyarrhythmia originating in an isolated ectopic atrial focus which fires at a rate of 250 to 350 beats per minute, with a ventricular response that is generally some specific ratio of atrial to ventricular beats, such as 4 to 1 or 2 to 1.

Rate: atrial and ventricular rates are not identical. Atrial rate is 250–350. Ventricular rate is some proportion of that.

Rhythm: generally ventricular rhythm is regular.

ECG Appearance: P wave is best visualized in leads II, III, AVF, where the P waves are discrete and separated by isoelectric intervals. The P wave is lost in a sawtooth pattern, but occurs in a regular interval. Because there is only one ectopic focus, the P waves all look identical, but since they do not originate in the SA node, they lack the normal rounded symmetrical appearance. The P wave has a relatively high voltage, and is sharp, asymmetrical, and pointed. An irritable focus in the walls of the atria overtakes the SA node as pacemaker. The AV node is unable to respond to each beat and therefore blocks many of these impulses, allowing every second, third, or fourth beat to reach the ventricle. Conduction from the AV node is normal, resulting in the normal appearance of the QRS (Fig. 5-5).

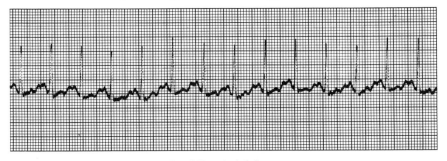

Fig. 5-5. Atrial flutter.

Cause: atrial flutter is rarely seen without pathology. It is most commonly encountered in patients with ischemic heart disease, valvular heart disease, acute myocardial infarction, hypoxia, emphysema, pulmonary embolus, congestive heart failure, pulmonary edema, hyperthyroidism.

Signs and Symptoms: patient describes palpitation and dyspnea. The pulse rate is regular and may not be rapid. The apical rate is higher than the pulse rate.

Clinical Significance: the heart loses its atrial kick, and the efficiency of the heart is reduced. With a rapid ventricular response circulation may be impaired.

Treatment: digitalis and oxygen. If cardiac or cerebral circulation is compromised, D-C cardioversion may be necessary.

Atrial Fibrillation

Atrial fibrillation is a tachyarrhythmia created by the firing of multiple ectopic foci in the atria. No impulse is able to depolarize the atria completely and only an occasional impulse is able to be conducted through the AV node.

Rate: atrial rate 350–600; ventricular rate 100–160.

Rhythm: irregularly irregular. Totally disorganized atrial electrical activity causes grossly irregular ventricular pattern. Many myofibrils are firing but none are able to create a contraction.

ECG Appearance: no apparent P waves. P waves appear only as an irregular baseline with occasional small shallow spikes. The P-R interval is not measurable. The QRS is of normal configuration and duration and occurs in an irregular transmission. Atrial fibrillation is best visualized in lead V_1. The feeble atrial contractions cause only small voltage changes, seen as an undulating baseline. The QRS response occurs in erratic fashion because the AV node is continually bombarded by impulses, many of which arrive while the node is refractory (Fig. 5-6).

Cause: coronary artery disease, hypertensive heart disease, rheumatic heart disease, hyperthyroidism, pericarditis, pulmonary embolus, neoplasia, post-operative thoracic surgery.

Signs and Symptoms: if the ventricular response is slow, the patient may be unaware of the irregularity. With a rapid ventricular response, the patient may describe palpitations. Apical and ventricle pulse rates are discrepant. The radial pulse will appear irregularly irregular.

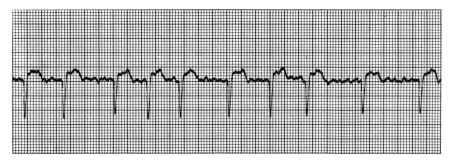

Fig. 5-6. Atrial fibrillation.

Clinical Significance: loss of atrial kick causes loss of cardiac efficiency of approximately 25 percent. At a rate of 150 or during exercise, cardiac output may be diminished by as much as 70 percent. Pre-load of the ventricles is increased and congestive heart failure may occur. Patients with chronic atrial fibrillation tend to develop thrombi. The ineffective beating of the atria causes blood to pool, leading to platelet aggregation and clot formation. Eventually the thrombus may dislodge, enter the arterial circulation, and cause cerebral vascular accidents and peripheral artery emboli. Thirty percent of all patients with chronic atrial fibrillation experience at least one embolic phenomenon. Atrial fibrillation decreases coronary blood flow by 35–40 percent and renal flow by 20 percent.[3]

Treatment: digitalis is the drug of choice. If symptoms are severe or congestive heart failure occurs, D-C cardioversion may be necessary.

AV Nodal Rhythm

AV nodal rhythm (Junctional Rhythm) is a rhythm created by the AV node, usually as a result of depressed SA nodal activity.

Rate: 40–60

Rhythm: regular; constant P-R interval

ECG Appearance: P wave is abnormal, usually inverted; may occur prior to, after, or be buried in the QRS complex. The QRS complex is of normal configuration and duration. The P wave is usually inverted in lead II, upright in AVR as a result of retrograde conduction.

Cause: digitalis toxicity, posterior wall infarction, ischemic heart disease

Signs and Symptoms: none

Clinical Significance: the slowed rate of atrial discharge allows other ectopic foci to take over. The AV node may become fatigued and fail to fire, leading to complete heart block and cardiac arrest.

Treatment: atropine or Isuprel

Nodal Tachycardia

AV nodal tachycardia is a rapid rhythm originating in the AV node.

Rate: 100–180

Rhythm: regular

ECG Appearance: P wave is abnormal in shape, usually being inverted. It may occur prior to or after the QRS complex. The QRS complex is of normal configuration and duration. A rapid focus in the AV junction usurps the SA node, causing retrograde depolarization of the atria with inversion of the P wave.

Cause: digitalis toxicity, posterior infarction

Signs and Symptoms: palpitations and dyspnea

Clinical Significance: rapid ventricular rate may predispose the patient to angina, congestive heart failure, or cerebral insufficiency.

Treatment: D-C cardioversion

First Degree Atrioventricular (AV) Block

AV block is an electrical block in the AV node which delays the passage of the wave of depolarization from the atria to the ventricles. In first degree block, the AV node delays the atrial impulse, creating a prolonged P-R interval. Once the AV node is stimulated, however, the conduction proceeds normally through the ventricles.

Rate: normal

Rhythm: regular

ECG Appearance: P wave is of normal configuration; there is one P wave for each QRS complex. The QRS complex is of normal configuration and duration. The singular characteristic of this dysrhythmia is a P-R interval prolonged beyond .20 seconds. But this prolonged P-R interval remains constant from beat to beat (Fig. 5-7).

Cause: digitalis toxicity, ischemic heart disease, rheumatic heart disease, hyperkalemia, posterior wall infarction.

Signs and Symptoms: none. Diagnosis by ECG only.

Clinical Significance: may represent injury to AV node; may be precursor of second or third degree heart block.

Treatment: none. Discontinue digitalis if it is the underlying culprit.

Second Degree AV Block: Wenckebach Phenomenon

Wenckebach Phenomenon is a second degree AV block characterized by a progressively increasing P-R interval.

Rate: atrial rate is normal but higher than the ventricular rate.

Rhythm: P waves are related to the QRS complex in a consistently repetitive manner. The P-R interval increases with each successive P wave until one P wave is blocked, and the cycle repeats itself.

ECG Appearance: P waves are of normal configuration but are more numerous than QRS complexes. The QRS complex is of normal configuration. The P-R interval lengthens between successive beats, and the R-R interval shortens. The pattern is predictable. The dropped beat is a P wave not followed by a QRS complex (Fig. 5-8).

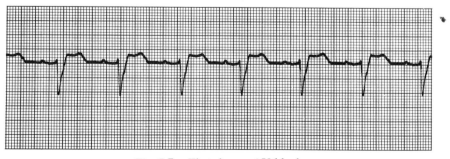

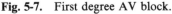

Fig. 5-7. First degree AV block.

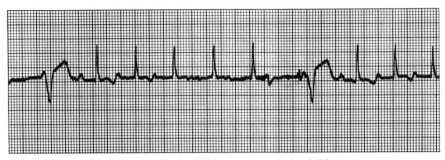

Fig. 5-8.   Second degree AV block: Wenckebach Phenomenon.

Cause: digitalis toxicity, ischemic heart disease, posterior wall infarction.

Signs and Symptoms: the patient usually is unaware of the reduced ventricular rate.

Clinical Significance: this block is usually transient but may progress into complete heart block.

Treatment: there is no means available for increasing conduction through the AV node, but atropine, Isuprel or epinephrine may be tried.

Second Degree AV Block: Mobitz II

Mobitz II is a rarer but more severe form of second degree heart block, typified by a series of non-conducted P waves followed by a P wave that is conducted normally.

Rate: atrial is normal; ventricular rate depends on the degree of block. P waves are more numerous than QRS complexes.

Rhythm: atrial is regular; ventricular rhythm varies with degree of block. P waves are consistently related to the ventricular beats.

ECG Appearance: P-R interval remains constant for conducted beats and may be normal or prolonged for non-conducted beats. The QRS occurs suddenly and may have a normal appearance.

Cause: acute infarction, ventricular septal defect, degenerative disease.

Signs and Symptoms: angina, cerebral insufficiency

Clinical Significance: severe arrhythmia which usually progresses to complete heart block with cardiac arrest.

Treatment: pacemaker

Third Degree or Complete Heart Block

None of the atrial impulses stimulate the AV node when a complete heart block exists. As a result, the unstimulated ventricle beats independently of the atria.

Rate: slow. Ventricular rate is less than 40. Atrial rate is normal or slow.

Rhythm: QRS rhythm is regular. P waves are regular. The P waves lack correlation to the QRS complexes.

ECG Appearance: P waves have a normal configuration. The P-R interval is completely variable. The QRS complex may be of normal configuration or abnormally wide, depending on the location of the ventricular focus.

Cause: anoxia is the primary pathology, although digitalis toxicity may cause the block.

Signs and Symptoms: if the ventricular rate is adequate to sustain circulation, symptoms may not develop. At slow rates, syncope or Stokes-Adams syndrome may occur as a result of inadequate cardiac output. Pulse rate will be 40 or less.

Clinical Significance: ventricular standstill may occur if the ventricles fatigue. Death ensues without a pacemaker.

Treatment: pacemaker.

Bundle Branch Block

The bundle branch block is characterized by a functional or anatomic discontinuity in a bundle branch which slows transmission of impulses through the ventricles. Because the ventricle normally supplied by the blocked bundle branch must be supplied by impulses traveling from the opposite ventricle through the intraventricular septum, the QRS complex is prolonged beyond .10 second. Additionally, because the ventricles do not depolarize simultaneously, there is a characteristic M or W shaped appearance to the complex.

Right Bundle Branch Block (RBBB)

Rate: normal

Rhythm: regular

ECG Appearance: P wave is normal in configuration and duration, and there is a P wave for each QRS. The P-R interval is normal. The QRS complex is widened beyond .12 seconds. The T wave deflection is opposite to that of the QRS complex. Lead V_1 shows a RSR' or M shaped complex. Lead V_6 shows a QRS or W shaped complex.

Cause: RBBB may be a normal pattern or it may occur as a result of underlying cardiac or pulmonary disease.

Signs and Symptoms: no clinical findings. A 12-lead ECG is necessary for diagnosis.

Clinical Significance: benign. Once it occurs the ECG rarely reverts to normal.

Left Bundle Branch Block (LBBB)

Rate: normal, but may be faster or slower than normal.

Rhythm: regular

ECG Appearance: P wave configuration and duration are normal. The P-R interval is normal. There is a P wave before each QRS complex. The QRS complex becomes widened and bizarre and the T wave is inverted. These changes are seen particularly well in the chest leads. Lead V_1 shows a QS complex. Lead V_6 shows a wide entirely positive R wave. The waves may show notching, and a characteristic W shaped complex occurs in V_1 and an M shaped complex in V_6.

Cause: LBBB is always associated with such serious heart disease as atherosclerotic heart disease, rheumatic heart disease, valvular heart disease, myocarditis, myocardial infarction, diptheria, primary or metastatic tumor.

Signs and Symptoms: none; however, LBBB does correlate significantly with cardiomegaly.

Clinical Significance: the arrhythmia itself is not serious. It does, however, indicate serious organic long-standing heart disease; therefore these patients should not be unduly stressed.

Treatment: none.

Premature Ventricular Contraction (PVC)

PVC is an impulse originating in the specialized conduction system of the ventricle below the site of bifurcation of the Bundle of His. This is the most common of all arrhythmias.

Rate: determined by the basic rate and number of PVCs.

Rhythm: variable. May be regular with exception of the premature beat; may be regularly irregular as in bigeminy, a condition which pairs a normal beat with a PVC; or may be irregularly irregular if PVCs are frequent and arise from many ectopic foci.

ECG Appearance: P wave is normal, but is not identifiable with the PVC since the impulse does not originate in the SA node or atrium. The P-R interval before the PVC is determined by whether the P wave is blocked, conducted normally, or activated in a retrograde fashion. The QRS complex is normal except for the PVC, when it becomes widened and bizarre in shape. The beats preceding and following the PVC are usually normal. The PVC will be followed by a compensatory pause. The time between the beat preceding and the beat following the PVC is equal to the time of two normal beats. The QRS has a high voltage. The T wave has a deflection opposite to that of the QRS (Fig. 5-9).

Cause: most common of rhythm disturbances; occurs in 62 percent of the population.[4] It can be caused by caffeine, alcohol, tobacco, anxiety. Can also be

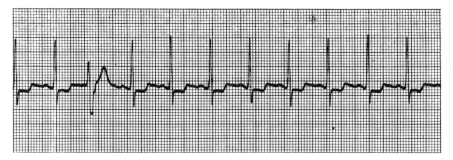

Fig. 5-9. Premature ventricular contraction.

drug induced in digitalis toxicity, hypokalemia, decreased serum calcium, epinephrine, Isuprel, aminophylline. Pathologic: hypoxia is the leading source of PVCs. Congestive heart failure, fever, infection, acidosis, anemia, mitral valve disease, and myocardial infarction may also be causes of ventricular irritability.

Signs and Symptoms: patients usually describe a "skipped beat," a surging sensation in the neck or throat. This sensation is due to the post-extrasystolic beat which empties ventricles that are overfilled because of the compensatory pause.

Clinical Significance: PVCs that occur infrequently are benign in the absence of heart disease. PVCs are considered on a scale of ventricular irritability. In ascending order of significance: occasional PVC; more than six PVCs per minute; paired PVCs or two in a row; multifocal PVCs or PVCs all of which differ in appearance, usually from multiple foci. PVCs may herald ventricular fibrillation, series of three uninterrupted PVCs, R on T phenomenon (PVCs that fall on the peak of the T wave of the preceding beat may cause ventricular tachycardia. The peak of the T wave is associated with a vulnerable period in the action potential, where less than normal stimuli may cause discharge). PVCs decrease coronary bloodflow by 12 percent and renal blood by 8 to 10 percent.[3]

Treatment: eliminate underlying cause: caffeine, tobacco, drugs. Administer oxygen to hypoxic patient. Patients with more than six PVCs a minute or greater signs of ventricular irritability are treated with Lidocaine.

Ventricular Tachycardia

By definition ventricular tachycardia is a run of three or more PVCs in a row. Ventricular tachycardia may occur in short bursts or may occur paroxysmally.

Rate: 100–250

Rhythm: regular or irregular

ECG Appearance: no apparent P wave, no R-R interval. The QRS is wide and bizarre (Fig. 5-10).

Cause: myocardial ischemia.

Signs and Symptoms: patients are immediately aware of the sudden rapid heart action and describe palpitation and dyspnea. The ventricles cannot fill sufficiently and this causes hypotension, angina, shock, congestive heart failure, pulmonary edema, cerebral and myocardial damage.

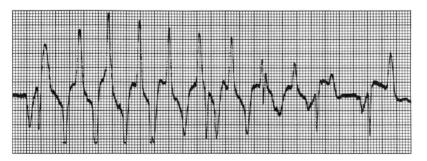

Fig. 5-10. Ventricular tachycardia.

Clinical Significance: Ventricular tachycardia is a precursor of ventricular fibrillation because rapid stimulation decreases the refractory period of the heart. Since cardiac output cannot be maintained, it is a life threatening arrhythmia. During ventricular tachycardia, coronary flow and renal flow decreases 60 percent.[3]

Treatment: D-C cardioversion, Lidocaine.

Ventricular Fibrillation

This arrythmia is created by many irritable foci in the ventricle, each firing at its own intrinsic rate, causing a chaotic twitching of the ventricles.

Rate: rapid, disorganized

Rhythm: irregular

ECG Appearance: P wave is not seen, the P-R interval is not seen, the QRS complexes are totally chaotic, with irregular oscillations that are not discernible.

Cause: exact cause is unknown.

Signs and Symptoms: patient loses consciousness without warning. The heartbeat is inaudible. Peripheral pulses are absent and cyanosis occurs. Blood pressure is not palpable, the pupils dilate, and convulsions occur.

Clinical Significance: if not reversed, death occurs within 3 minutes. During ventricular fibrillation coronary and cerebral blood flow is negligible.

Treatment: D-C cardioversion.

Acute Myocardial Infarction

An acute myocardial infarction is heralded by the presence of a significant Q wave. A significant Q wave is at least .04 second in width or 1/3 the size of the QRS complex. Omit lead AVR when looking for the presence of significant Q waves. Associated with the presence of Q waves are ST segment elevation and tall T waves. This is an immediate effect of an acute infarction and evolves within hours. These findings occur because of changes in myocardial depolarization and repolarization.

These signs are found in the leads that are parallel to the damage and whose positive terminal is closest to the infarction. Therefore an anterior wall infarction would be indicated by Q waves and ST segment elevation in the chest leads V_1, V_2, V_3, V_4. In an anteroseptal infarction there is loss of the R in V_1 and V_2, resulting in a completely negative QS complex in leads V_5, V_6. When changes occur in leads II, III, and AVF, an inferior wall infarction is suspected. Similarly, Q waves in leads I, AVL, and V_5, V_6 are strongly suggestive of a lateral wall infarction.

The most difficult infarction to determine is a posterior wall infarction, since this surface of the ventricles does not face the positive terminal of any of the 12 conventional leads. Therefore reciprocal changes, a tall R wave and ST segment depression in leads V_1 and V_2, are suggestive of a posterior infarction.

Differential Diagnoses

P Wave. The P Wave is normally symmetrical and round: .08 to .12 seconds in duration, and .1 to .3 mv in amplitude. Normal lead deflections are as follows: I, upright; II, upright; III, any; AVR, inverted; AVL, any; AVF, upright; V_1–V_6, upright. If P waves are present and normal in shape, size, and configuration, the originating stimulus is the SA node.

Inversion in AVF, I, and II, and upright in AVR, indicates retrograde conduction and probable nodal rhythm. Increased amplitude indicates atrial hypertrophy especially associated with valve disease, hypertension, cor pulmonale, and congenital heart disease. Increased width indicates left atrial enlargement. A diphasic P wave is an important sign of left atrial enlargement when the second half of the P wave is significantly negative in III or V_1.

When the left atrium is mainly involved (mitral disease), P waves become wide and notched. The P wave is taller in I than in III. Notching is significant when the distance between peaks exceeds .04 seconds in duration. A tall, pointed P wave taller in III than in I indicates right atrial enlargement. Absent P waves indicate sinus node block or AV nodal rhythm.

QRS Complex. The QRS complex can show a variable pattern in I, II, III, AVF, AVL. It is usually inverted in AVR. In the precordial leads the R wave becomes progressively larger from V_1 to V_6, and the S wave becomes progressively smaller.

A widened QRS with RSR′ in V_1 may indicate right bundle branch block. A widened QS in V_1 may indicate left bundle branch block. A widened bizarre QRS complex without a P wave preceding it, and with the T wave opposite in direction to the QRS with a compensatory pause, is usually a PVC.

An abnormally tall R in V_1 associated with an abnormally deep S in V_6 (equal to or greater than 35 mv), and an R in AVL greater than 13 mv, indicates left ventricular hypertrophy. A larger R wave in V_1, of normal duration, indicates right ventricular hypertrophy.

ST Segment. Elevation is the earliest sign of myocardial infarction. Look for concomitant Q wave. Transient elevation with angina indicates Prinzmetal angina. Persistent elevation following an infarction indicates ventricular aneurysm. Elevation with low voltage complex indicates pericarditis. It may also be a normal variant.[5]

Depression with squared off shape is indicative of subendocardial infarction. A scooping U shaped segment is indicative of digitalis toxicity. A sharp, pointed depression indicates hypokalemia, while a down-sloping or horizontal ST segment during stress tests indicates a positive test.[5]

T Wave Inversion. Normally inverted T waves in leads with negative QRS, such as AVR, may also be inverted in V_1 and V_2, indicating an evolving phase of transmural myocardial infarction. Sharp inversion indicates evolving phase of pericarditis. T wave inversion in right chest leads is produced by RBBB; in left chest leads, by LBBB. T wave inversion may occur with tachycardia, mitral valve prolapse, and subarachnoid hemorrhage.

Tall T Wave. A tall T wave is found in patients with hyperkalemia, and is seen in myocardial ischemia without infarction in patients with cerebral vascular accidents.

Non-specific ST-T Wave Changes. This expression refers to ST segment depression less than 1 mm with T wave flattening or slight T wave inversion. These are abnormal changes but are not specific indicators of ischemia. They may be due to ischemic heart disease, drugs, hyperventilation, infection, electrolyte imbalance, and pulmonary disease.

Bradyarrhythmias. There are four main causes of slow rates:

1. Sinus bradycardia: each QRS is preceded by a P wave and the P is negative in AVR, upright in II.

2. Nodal rhythm: characterized by a P wave that is conducted in a retrograde manner, manifested by an upright P in AVR and an inverted P in II, or a P wave that is not seen.

3. Second or third degree block: dropped beats are seen on the rhythm strip.

4. Atrial fibrillation with slow ventricular response: ECG shows characteristic fibrillation waves.[5]

Tachyarrhythmias. Tachyarrhythmias should be diagnosed as follows:

1. Paroxysmal atrial tachycardia (PAT): rapid and absolutely regular rhythm; P wave not always discernible. Patient will describe sudden onset; returns to normal sinus rhythm with carotid sinus massage.

2. Sinus tachycardia: P wave precedes each QRS.

3. Atrial fibrillation: characterized by a wavy, undulating baseline with poorly discernible P waves and irregular ventricular response.

4. Atrial flutter: characterized by a sawtooth pattern and a QRS that occurs in a predictable manner.

5. Ventricular tachycardia: characterized by wide, bizarre QRS complexes and no apparent P waves.

CONCLUSION

Knowledge of ECG interpretation will enhance the ability of the physical therapist to interpret chart records, to communicate with other health professionals concerning cardiac patients, and to identify abnormal ECG responses which may occur during physical therapy treatments.

REFERENCES

1. James TN: Anatomy of the conduction system of the heart. In: The Heart, ed. Hurst JW. New York, McGraw-Hill, 1978
2. James TN: Anatomy of the coronary arteries and veins. In: The Heart, ed. Hurst JW. New York, McGraw-Hill, 1978

3. Corday E, Lang T-W: Altered physiology associated with cardiac arrhythmias. In: The Heart, ed. Hurst JW. New York, McGraw-Hill, 1978
4. Marriott HJL, Myersburg RJ: Recognition and treatment of cardiac arrhythmias and conduction disturbances. In: The Heart, ed. Hurst JW. New York, McGraw-Hill, 1978
5. Goldberger AL, Goldberger E: Clinical Electrocardiography: A Simplified Approach. St Louis, CV Mosby, 1977

6 | Progressive Exercise Tolerance Testing

R.G. McAllister, Jr.
Stuart L. Lowenthal

Progressive exercise tolerance testing is a simple, safe, and reliable procedure for patient evaluation.[1-4] It involves such familiar, nonthreatenting activity as treadmill walking or pedalling a bicycle ergometer. Continuous electrocardiographic (ECG) monitoring allows early detection of potential cardiac difficulties, often before symptoms occur. The use of standardized protocols permits accurate and reproducible evaluation of exercise capacity, and exercise-induced ECG changes are clearly related to the presence of coronary arterial disease as well as to patient prognosis. Over the past decade, exercise testing has become one of the most useful procedures in the evaluation of patients, and is clearly applicable in smaller community hospital settings.[5, 6]

Because the facilities required for exercise testing are minimal, we believe that a diagnostic exercise laboratory should be as available as routine clinical laboratory resources in the hospital environment. A small area of space, a motorized treadmill, and an ECG monitoring unit form the basis for an exercise laboratory. A single therapist, trained in exercise testing methodology, can carry out the entire procedure, with a licensed physician physically present in the area. The graded exercise stress test (GXT) itself requires a total time of 30 to 60 minutes, including patient preparation and recovery.

Indications for exercise testing[3, 4] are outlined in Table 6-1 and reviewed in detail in succeeding sections.

Table 6-1. Indications for exercise testing

1. Evaluation of chest pain syndromes
2. Evaluation for exercise-induced dysrhythmias
3. Evaluation and quantitation of functional capacity
4. Evaluation of efficacy of drug therapy
5. Evaluation of efficacy of non-pharmacologic therapy
6. Screening for ischemic heart disease
7. Research in exercise physiology

THE GXT AS A DIAGNOSTIC PROCEDURE

Ischemic Heart Disease

Exercise testing is most frequently used for the diagnostic evaluation of patients thought to have coronary, or ischemic, heart disease.[1-9] These patients may have such symptoms as chest pain, or may be asymptomatic but have a sufficiently impressive coronary risk factor profile to justify GXT evaluation.[10] In either case, an understanding of the pathophysiology of myocardial ischemia will make clear this use of exercise testing.

Myocardial ischemia occurs when blood flow through the coronary arterial circulation is inadequate to meet the oxygen needs of the cardiac muscle. The supply of blood (and, therefore, oxygen) is largely determined by the presence or absence of disease in the coronary arteries. When proximal atherosclerotic lesions produce significant degrees of lumenal narrowing, restriction of coronary flow will result. Although blood flow may be adequate at rest, increasing myocardial oxygen need, such as occurs with exercise, in the presence of compromised flow will result in an imbalance between oxygen supply and demand, producing the symptoms and signs of myocardial ischemia.

The major factors that determine myocardial oxygen demand include systolic arterial pressure, left ventricular size, heart rate, and contractility.[11] Of these, heart rate is most easily monitored. In normal subjects, heart rate accurately reflects both coronary blood flow and myocardial oxygen demand.[12, 13] Therefore, heart rate is monitored during exercise testing as an estimate of the amount of work done by the heart for a given amount of exercise. If coronary atherosclerotic disease is present and myocardial ischemia occurs during the GXT, it is seen reproducibly at the same heart rate in each exercise session, provided the conditions of testing are similar.

These observations provide the basis for exercise testing procedures based on heart rate increases. Older procedures, such as the Master Test,[14] are load-standardized, in that the patient is required to do a fixed amount of work. In some patients, the fixed work load may be inadequate to elicit evidence of ischemia; in others, the load may be excessive.[15] Diagnostic accuracy is clearly improved when the patient's exercise load is gradually and progressively increased, allowing detection of symptoms (such as chest pain) or ECG signs to herald the onset of myocardial ischemia and permitting the GXT to be halted at that point.

The ECG must be continuously monitored throughout the exercise test pro-

PRE - EXERCISE

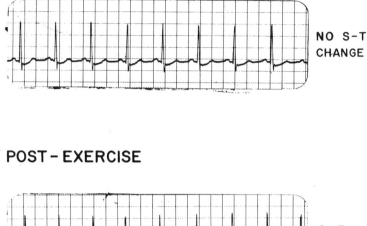

NO S-T
CHANGE

POST - EXERCISE

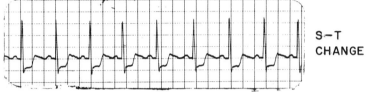

S-T
CHANGE

Fig. 6-1. This illustration shows representative samples of lead V_5 before and after exercise. Note the marked depression in the ST segment produced by exercise testing; this is characteristic of an ischemic response.

cedure. Myocardial ischemia is most accurately diagnosed when *both* chest pain and typical ECG changes occur.[16] The chest pain is typically anginal, being usually substernal, associated with dyspnea, and progressively severe as exercise continues. ECG changes occur in the ST segment of the electrocardiogram, as shown in Figure 6-1, and usually precede the onset of symptoms. Both chest pain and ECG changes tend to resolve rapidly when exercise is stopped and the heart rate falls. Nitroglycerine tablets for sublingual use must always be at hand in the GXT laboratory and should be given to any patient whose ischemia does not resolve within 2 to 3 minutes after ending exercise.

When the GXT results in chest pain and ST segment depression on the ECG, there is a high degree of correlation with evidence for proximal coronary arterial obstruction at angiography.[16, 17] When ischemia occurs at relatively low levels of exercise, significant coronary artery obstruction will be found in at least 85 to 90 percent of subjects. In addition, the results of GXT procedures accurately predict the likelihood of subsequent "coronary events," including myocardial infarction.[7, 18]

The sensitivity and specificity of GXT procedures depend upon a number of factors. First, the population of subjects studied is important. In patients who are thought likely to have ischemic heart disease because of chest pain symptoms or an impressive coronary risk factor profile, the GXT is particularly accurate.[19-21]

In asymptomatic subjects, however, a significant number of false-positive tests will occur, leading to potential difficulties when the GXT is used as a screening procedure.[10, 22]

Second, the ECG criteria used are important in determining both sensitivity and specificity for the GXT. The most satisfactory combination results from a definition of "ischemic changes" as a flat or downsloping ST segment, depressed at least 1.0 mm below the baseline, and lasting for at least 0.08 seconds beyond the J-point.[1, 3, 23, 24] As the degree of ST segment depression increases, the sensitivity of the test increases.[25] Conversely, lesser degrees of ST segment shift decrease the specificity of the GXT as a diagnostic tool, and the evidence of false-positive results increases. Elevation of the ST segment indicates either acute, severe ischemia[26] or dyskinetic ventricular myocardium; if accompanied by chest pain, the GXT should be halted immediately.

Third, the sensitivity and specificity of the GXT are both diminished when conditions which predispose to false-positive results[22, 27–29] are not vigorously excluded (Table 6-2). Most patients taking digitalis, for instance, will have significant ST segment depression during exercise, not necessarily related to the presence or absence of ischemia, as a result of the drug's effects. Our laboratory interprets such tests as "nondiagnostic," indicating that the specificity of the GXT under such conditions is sufficiently low that a dependable diagnosis cannot be made with it (see Figs. 6-2, 6-3). In addition, sex seems to be an important factor in the specificity of the GXT, as the incidence of false-positive responses in normal women is sufficiently high that the usefulness of the GXT for women has been questioned.[30–32]

Of particular relevance to the troubling problem of nondiagnostic test results is the recent combination of GXT procedures with radioisotope administration.[33] Radioisotopic thallium is most widely used at this time, with administration of the substance at the end of symptom-limited exercise. The principle underlying this approach is that the tracer is distributed to the myocardium in proportion to the degree of blood flow; focal areas of decreased tracer concentration indicate decreased coronary flow and, presumably, myocardial ischemia.[34] This procedure appears now to be a reasonably reliable and accurate method for the noninvasive detection of ischemia, and particularly useful in patients likely to have false-positive results by conventional ECG criteria.[35]

Other recent efforts have involved increasingly sophisticated computer pro-

Table 6-2. Conditions associated with ECG changes during exercise testing which simulate ischemic responses (false-positive GXT)

1. Wolff-Parkinson-White ECG pattern
2. Left bundle branch block
3. Left ventricular hypertrophy
4. Hypokalemia
5. Digitalis and/or estrogen administration
6. Resting abnormalities of the ST segment

FALSE + EXERCISE STRESS TEST: 49 y/o man with LVH

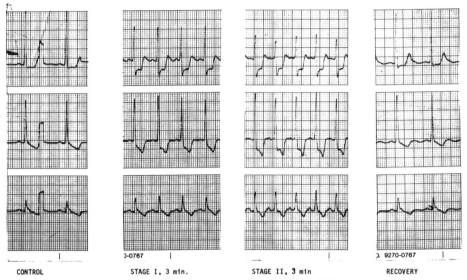

CONTROL   STAGE I, 3 min.   STAGE II, 3 min   RECOVERY

Fig. 6-2. Representative samples of leads V_4 (top), V_5 (middle), and V_6 (bottom) are shown before, during, and after exercise in a patient with left ventricular hypertrophy (LVH). The pre-GXT ECG is clearly abnormal, as shown by ST depression and T inversion in the control tracing. With exercise, increased ST depression occurred. No chest pain was reported by the patient. Coronary arteriography was normal. This, then, is a false-positive ECG response to exercise.

grams for interpretation of the exercise ECG; the resources required, however, are presently unavailable outside larger teaching centers.[36]

Evaluation of Dysrhythmias

The GXT may be particularly useful in eliciting tachyrhythmias which are suspected by a history of palpitations and/or syncope, but which are not detected by the resting ECG. When the arrhythmia occurs, a proper diagnosis may be made and, if indicated, specific antiarrhythmic therapy prescribed. Exercise-induced ventricular arrhythmias are particularly hazardous and may result from an ischemic focus.[37-39] Ambulatory ECG monitoring has, in most studies, provided better detection of suspected arrhythmias than the GXT.[37, 40] However, certain advantages are associated with use of the GXT: as opposed to the Holter monitoring procedure, the physician is present when the arrhythmia occurs and treatment may be initiated promptly; in addition, drug efficacy can be evaluated after beginning therapy by repeating the GXT, after the patient has been treated, to determine if the previously-elicited dysrhythmia has been suppressed adequately; finally, an evaluation of the patient's exercise capacity can be derived from the GXT procedure. If, on the other hand, the suspected dysrhythmia is not elicited

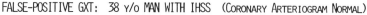

FALSE-POSITIVE GXT: 38 y/o MAN WITH IHSS (Coronary Arteriogram Normal)

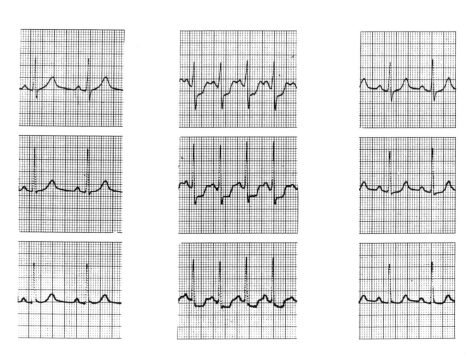

CONTROL   6 MIN EXERCISE   RECOVERY

Fig. 6-3.   Representative samples of leads V_4, V_5, and V_6 are shown before, during, and after exercise in a patient with a normal control ECG. Marked ST depression without chest pain occurred with exertion. Angiographic study revealed normal coronary arteries, but IHSS (idiopathic hypertrophic subaortic stenosis) was present. This is an example of a false-positive GXT in which the pre-exercise ECG was normal.

by GXT, ambulatory monitoring for prolonged periods of time can be subsequently carried out. Optimal detection of suspected rhythm disturbances is usually found by a combination of GXT and subsequent ambulatory monitoring.[40]

Because of the ever-present possibility of potentially lethal tachyarrhythmias during a GXT, personnel should be trained in cardiac resuscitative procedures, and an emergency cart with defibrillator and the appropriate drugs and equipment should be available in the exercise laboratory.

Heart rate normally increases during progressive exercise until symptoms due to disease or fatigue indicate that the procedure should be halted. If the heart rate increase is considerably less than normally seen, chronotropic incompetence exists and may be associated with a grave prognosis, usually from ischemic complications.[7] Many drugs may prevent normal increases in heart rate with exercise, including beta-blockers and sympatholytic agents used in antihypertensive therapy. A pre-GXT history is important to determine if such drugs are being administered, as evaluation of the heart rate response to exercise stress cannot be made in their presence.

THE GXT IN EVALUATION OF FUNCTIONAL CAPACITY

The GXT is a standard tool in the evaluation of functional capacity[41] (Table 6-1). It may be used to determine if a patient's complaints of weakness or easy fatigability are valid, and it allows comparison with standards of performance in comparable age- and sex-matched populations, both trained and untrained. Furthermore, the GXT is a useful procedure for sedentary individuals who anticipate beginning an exercise program; it allows detection of ischemic changes unsuspected because of the subject's lethargic lifestyle,[10] as well as evaluation for exercise-related arrhythmias,[32] and permits an exercise prescription to be individually compiled by the therapist.[6, 42]

The usefulness of the GXT in evaluation of functional capacity depends upon selection of a standard protocol for exercise test procedures and rigid adherence to the requirements of that protocol. A number of different regimens for treadmill testing have been developed and intensively studied: each has certain advantages and disadvantages, which have been recently reviewed. Perhaps the most widely used protocol is that developed by Bruce and his associates;[1] it has the advantages of requiring relatively little time to perform, being applicable for evaluation of subjects over a wide age range, and having nomograms available for estimates of comparative performance by a given subject.

Use of the Bruce protocol (Table 6-3) allows estimation for an individual subject of the functional aerobic impairment (FAI) by comparison with published nomograms;[41] the FAI is the difference between the observed maximal oxygen intake (or, maximum exercise tolerance) and that expected for a healthy person of similar age and sex. This is a useful way to compare a specific patient's performance with those found in a reference population.

Although reference nomograms published by Bruce et al use the FAI concept, other data are available which allow expression of GXT results as "metabolic equivalents" (MET). A MET is defined as resting oxygen consumption, usually 3.5 ml $O_2 \cdot kg^{-1} \cdot min^{-1}$. This term has found popularity with many exercise therapists and may be conceptually useful as a simplification of more cumbersome terms. Other chapters describe in detail the derivation of the MET and

Table 6-3. Bruce protocol for exercise testing

Stage	Treadmill Speed (mph)	Treadmill Elevation (% grade)	Energy Cost (METs)	Time (min)
1	1.7	10	5.1	3
2	2.5	12	7.1	3
3	3.4	14	10.0	3
4	4.2	16	14.0	3
5	5.0	18	15.7	3

other, similar approaches to quantitation of exercise capacity. A comparison between the various exercise testing protocols and oxygen uptake required for each level of exercise can be found in the recent paper by Fortuin and Weiss.[4]

It is important to remember that use of FAI or MET terms depends upon an exercise effort that is truly maximal, termed "symptom-limited" exercise testing. Submaximal exercise testing does not truly define a patient's maximum exercise capacity. The subject, prior to beginning the GXT, must appreciate the importance of a genuine effort to complete as much of the exercise protocol as possible. Most problems with patient compliance in this regard can be eliminated with satisfactory pre-test explanations.

When a standard protocol (such as the Bruce regimen) is used, the total time a subject can exercise serves as a good estimate of the efficacy of various therapeutic interventions. Serial GXT studies can determine objectively the adequacy of pharmacologic treatment in patients with ischemic heart disease and exercise

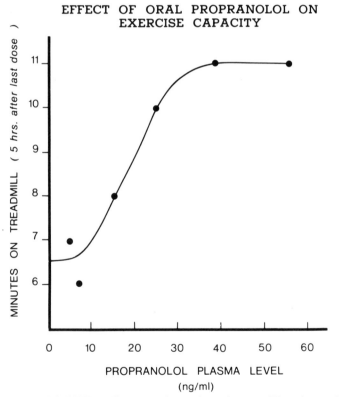

Fig. 6-4.   Use of serial GXT studies to evaluate drug therapy. The plasma level of propranolol, a beta-blocking drug, was increased by giving progressively larger doses, and serial GXT studies were carried out. When the patient's total exercise tolerance time was maximally increased (at a level of 30–40 ng/ml), the drug dose producing this optimal therapeutic result was administered chronically.

performance limited by angina pectoris. An example is shown in Figure 6-4, which relates the plasma level of propranolol (Inderal), a beta-adrenoceptor blocking drug, to exercise capacity, as reflected in total treadmill exercise time with the Bruce protocol, in a patient with symptomatic angina. As the dose of the drug was increased, plasma levels also increased, providing increasing therapeutic protection; a critical level for this patient was in the 30 to 40 ng/ml range, above which no further increase in exercise capacity occurred. Serial studies in this patient, therefore, defined the most appropriate drug dose for control of his symptoms. Similar approaches have been used for evaluation of nitrate therapy in angina, for evaluation of antiarrhythmic drug efficacy,[43, 44] and for determination of the effects of nonpharmacologic therapy.

With serial GXT studies, exercise training, as used in cardiac rehabilitation programs, can be shown to increase functional capacity (Fig. 6-5), independent of changes in drug treatment.[6, 45, 46] The GXT procedure is first used to define the

EFFECT OF TRAINING ON EXERCISE TOLERANCE

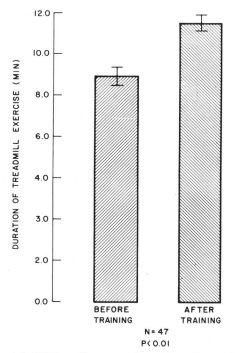

Fig. 6-5.   Use of serial GXT studies to evaluate the effects of exercise training. Forty-seven patients with ischemic heart disease underwent a 3-month period of exercise-based rehabilitation therapy. The mean exercise tolerance for the group prior to training was significantly less than that found after training ($p < 0.01$). Total exercise time during the Bruce protocol was used here as a reflection of functional capacity.

limits of exercise and heart rate increase which an individual patient can safely tolerate; an exercise prescription is then derived, under which a patient will exercise at a level producing a degree of heart rate increase shown to be safe for him during the GXT. Repeated GXT evaluations are useful in demonstrating the progressive improvement in functional capacity which results from exercise training; additionally, they provide a helpful psychologic boost by allowing the patient to see objective comparisons of his performance.

THE EXERCISE LABORATORY

Physical facilities required for an exercise laboratory include adequate space for a treadmill and an examination table or bed; an ECG monitoring unit with a recorder and oscilloscope; and an emergency cart with defibrillator and resuscitation equipment.[6] Additional space should be available in which patients can disrobe in privacy. Space for a waiting room is also useful.

The treadmill should have variable speed and elevation controls, allowing gradual alterations in either or both parameters during treadmill walking. Bicycle ergometers are used in Europe but are less popular in this country since bicycle exercise is less familiar to Americans than walking. There are differences between bicycle and treadmill exercise, with the former providing greater stress on the cardiovascular system for any given oxygen uptake level.[47]

Many laboratories use a single-channel ECG monitoring system to detect arrhythmias and ischemic ST changes induced by exercise, although considerably more complex instrumentation is available and aggressively advertised. Sensitivity of the GXT in detection of ischemic changes is enhanced by the use of multiple leads during exercise testing;[48] if a single lead is monitored, the most satisfactory is the V_5 lead or a bipolar approximation of V_5, such as the CC_5 lead.[49] In addition, the response of arterial pressure to exercise must be monitored, since a fall in blood pressure with exercise is an indication of impaired left ventricular function.[50] A standard sphygmomanometer and stethoscope are adequate for this purpose, although, again, more complex devices are available. Emergency carts are usually standardized with AHA recommendations by selected hospital committees, and must include a defibrillator unit checked at intervals to assure proper performance.

Bruce recommends that patients undergoing GXT procedures sign a statement giving informed consent.[2] Such a statement should define the purpose, the risks, the potential benefits, and the precautions taken to assure the patient's benefit.

The individual responsible for carrying out GXT procedures should be adequately trained in ECG interpretation to recognize abnormalities in rhythm and ischemic ECG changes. Familiarity with the protocols selected for use and the available resuscitation equipment is essential. Since physical therapists are specifically trained in exercise physiology, are familiar with hospital environments, and are experienced in patient relations, we feel that the physical therapist is the proper individual to develop and direct an exercise laboratory. A licensed physician should be present during each GXT procedure, in the event medical expertise is needed; the physician need not be trained in exercise testing, and, in fact, need not play any role in the procedures when an experienced therapist is directing the GXT.[5] Interpretation of the exercise test should be relegated to a physician experienced in electrocardiography and in exercise physiology.

The exercise stress test itself is a procedure best learned by experience, as the primary variables are those introduced by different patients and their problems. A number of specific points should be followed, however, both to ensure the quality of the studies done and to avoid exposing test subjects to increased hazards. Prior to the GXT, care should be taken to exclude patients in whom the GXT procedure itself is contraindicated; a review of the clinical history, physical exam, and resting 12-lead ECG should suffice (Table 6-4). In addition, information should be obtained from the patient regarding current drug treatment, in order to determine if potential for false-positive test results is present (Table 6-2). The patient should have the details of the procedure explained, and treadmill walking should be demonstrated. Blood pressure should be recorded supine and standing prior to the test, at least once during each exercise stage, and each minute during post-GXT recovery. Similarly, a recording of the monitored ECG lead should be made at specified intervals throughout the procedure, as well as spontaneously as needed to record vital data on arrhythmias or ischemic changes.

The GXT should be halted when the information for which the procedure is done becomes apparent, or when symptoms and/or fatigue force the patient to stop. End-points for stress tests should be carefully reviewed and scrupulously observed (Table 6-5). Many protocols recommend that the patient stand briefly on the treadmill after the GXT for measurement of blood pressure and ECG recording, then return to a supine position on the examining table. Observation and monitoring should continue for at least 6 minutes, or for sufficient time to allow all symptoms to resolve, the ECG to return to normal, and heart rate and blood pressure to return to pre-GXT levels.

Table 6-4. Contraindications to exercise stress testing

Absolute Contraindications
1. Unstable ischemic heart disease
   a. Myocardial infarction within 3 weeks
   b. Recent onset of chest pain which may be angina
   c. Increase in frequency or severity of previously stable angina
2. Poorly controlled cardiac failure
3. Inadequately controlled hypertension
4. Serious arrhythmias at rest
   a. Uncontrolled atrial fibrillation or flutter
   b. Ventricular arrhythmias at rest, including bigeminy, ventricular couplets, and/or runs of ventricular tachycardia (3 or more VPB's in succession)
5. Acute illnesses which compromise treadmill performance
6. Neurological or orthopedic problems which preclude treadmill exercise

Relative Contraindications
1. Aortic outflow tract obstruction (valvular or subvalvular)
2. Severe pulmonary hypertension
3. Thyrotoxicosis
4. Patient reluctance to undergo procedure

Table 6-5. End-points for exercise stress testing

Objective
1. Absolute
   a. Fall in systolic blood pressure (over 20 mm Hg) with progressive exercise
   b. Rise in systolic blood pressure to potentially hazardous levels (over 250 mm Hg)
   c. Development of sustained atrial tachyarrhythmias
   d. Ventricular tachycardia
   e. Occurrence of second or third degree AV block
   f. Inability to walk effectively on the treadmill
2. Relative
   a. ST segment depression greater than 2.0 mm without chest pain or dyspnea

Subjective
1. Chest pain of increasing severity
2. Claudication
3. Dyspnea
4. Dizziness
5. Profound fatigue

Interpretation of the GXT is best carried out by the physician present at the procedure, provided he is trained in exercise testing. Alternatively, the recorded ECG strips and the data sheets compiled by the therapist can be interpreted later by an appropriately skilled consultant.

When proper patient exclusion is carried out, proper facilities are available, proper endpoints are observed, and progressive exercise protocols with constant ECG monitoring are used, the GXT is a safe procedure. Rochmis and Blackburn[51] reviewed 170,000 exercise tests in 73 medical centers in 1971, finding only 6 deaths occurring within one hour of the GXT. In almost 4,000 GXT procedures at the Good Samaritan Hospital in Lexington, we have seen only one major complication: a young man with recent onset chest pain, who should have been classified as "unstable ischemic heart disease," was subjected to vigorous exercise, and at a heart rate of 140/min developed severe chest pain; an acute myocardial infarction evolved. The patient is alive and well five years later.

CONCLUSIONS AND SUMMARY

Over the past 15 years, progressive exercise tolerance testing has become an established procedure for the evaluation of patients with cardiovascular disease; it is necessary for the objective determination of functional capacity. It is a valuable resource in the study of patients for cardiac rhythm disorders, especially when combined with ambulatory ECG monitoring. Finally, exercise testing is useful in determination of the efficacy of various therapeutic interventions, whether pharmacologic or surgical, or based on exercise training.

The GXT is a safe procedure when standards are followed. We feel that an exercise laboratory should be available in most hospital settings, at least in those which provide physical therapy resources. The physical therapist, trained in exercise physiology and experienced with patients, is the logical individual to develop and direct a hospital's exercise laboratory. The physical therapist should be specifically skilled in the interpretation of various aspects of exercise tolerance and can most effectively provide exercise advice and prescriptions for patients requiring exercise-based training and rehabilitation programs.

REFERENCES

1. Bruce RA, Hornsten TR: Exercise stress testing in evaluation of patients with ischemic heart disease. Prog Cardiovasc Dis 11:371–390, 1969
2. Bruce RA: Exercise testing of patients with coronary heart disease. Principles and normal standards for evaluation. Ann Clin Res 3:323–332, 1971
3. Blomqvist CG: Use of exercise testing for diagnostic and functional evaluation of patients with arteriosclerotic heart disease. Circulation 44:1120–1136, 1971
4. Fortuin NJ, Weiss JL: Exercise stress testing. Circulation 56:699–712, 1977
5. Lowenthal SL, McAllister RG: The use of exercise in diagnosis and treatment of cardiac patients in a community hospital: experience over 27 months. J Ky Med Assoc 74:171–176, 1976
6. Lowenthal SL, McAllister RG: Program for cardiac patients: stress testing and training. Phys Ther 56:1117–1123, 1976
7. Ellestad MH, Wan MKC: Predictive implications of stress testing. Follow-ups of 2,700 subjects after maximum treadmill stress testing. Circulation 51:363–369, 1975
8. Theroux P, Waters DD, Halphen C, et al: Prognostic value of exercise testing soon after myocardial infarction. N Engl J Med 301:341–345, 1979
9. McNeer JF, Margolis JR, Lee KL, et al: The role of the exercise test in the evaluation of patients for ischemic heart disease. Circulation 57:64–70, 1978
10. Bruce RA, McDonough JR: Stress testing in screening for cardiovascular disease. Bull NY Acad Med 45:1288–1297, 1969
11. Sonnenblick EH, Ross J Jr, Braunwald E: Oxygen consumption of the heart: newer concepts of its multifactorial determination. Am J Cardiol 22:328–333, 1968
12. Kitamura K, Jorgensen CR, Gobel FL, et al: Hemodynamic correlates of myocardial oxygen consumption during upright exercise. J Appl Physiol 32:516–520, 1972
13. Nelson RR, Gobel RL, Jorgensen CR, et al: Hemodynamic predictors of myocardial oxygen consumption during static and dynamic exercise. Circulation 50:1179–1185, 1974
14. Master AM: The two-step test of myocardial function. Am Heart J 10:495–501, 1935
15. Rowell LB, Taylor HL, Simonson E, Carlson WS: The physiologic fallacy of adjusting for body weight in performance of the Master two-step test. Am Heart J 70:461–464, 1965
16. Cole JP, Ellestad MH: Significance of chest pain during treadmill exercise: correlation with coronary events. Am J Cardiol 41:227–232, 1978
17. Goldschlager N, Selzer A, Cohn K: Treadmill stress tests as indicators of presence and severity of coronary artery disease. Ann Intern Med 85:277–282, 1976
18. Aronow WS: Thirty-month follow-up of maximal treadmill stress test and double Master's test in normal subjects. Circulation 47:287–290, 1973
19. Piessens J, Mieghem WV, Kesteloot H, de Geest H: Diagnostic value of clinical history, exercise testing, and atrial pacing in patients with chest pain. Am J Cardiol 33:351–356, 1974
20. Fabian J, Stolz I, Janota M, Rohac J: Reproducibility of exercise tests in patients with symptomatic ischemic heart disease. Br Heart J 37:785–789, 1975
21. Ellestad MH, Halliday WK: Stress testing in the prognosis and management of ischemic heart disease. Angiology 28:149–159, 1977

22. Weiner DA, Ryan TJ, McCabe CH, et al: Exercise stress testing. Correlations among history of angina, ST segment response, and prevalence of coronary artery disease in the coronary artery surgery study. N Engl J Med 301:230–235, 1979
23. Simonson E: Electrocardiographic stress tolerance tests. Prog Cardiovasc Dis 13:269–285, 1970
24. Sheffield LT, Reeves TJ: Graded exercise in the diagnosis of angina pectoris. Mod Concepts Cardiovasc Dis 34:1–5, 1965
25. Goldman S, Teslos S, Cohn K: Marked depth of ST depression during treadmill exercise testing. Chest 69:729–773, 1976
26. Fortuin NJ, Friesinger GC: Exercise-induced ST segment elevation: clinical, electrocardiographic, and arteriographic studies in 12 patients. Am J Med 49:459–464, 1970
27. Linhart JW, Turnoff HB: Pitfalls in diagnostic and functional evaluation using exercise testing. Chest 65:364–366, 1974
28. Surawicz B, Saito T: Exercise testing for detection of myocardial ischemia in patients with abnormal electrocardiograms at rest. Am J Cardiol 41:943–951, 1978
29. Surawicz B: Pitfalls in interpretation of ECG stress tests. Postgrad Med 65:54–69, 1979
30. Cumming GR, Dufresne C, Kich L, Samm J: Exercise electrocardiogram patterns in normal women. Br Heart J 35:1055–1061, 1973
31. Sketch MH, Mohiuddin SM, Lynch JD, et al: Significant sex differences in the correlation of electrocardiographic exercise testing and coronary arteriograms. Am J Cardiol 36:169–173, 1975
32. Jaffe MD: Effect of estrogens on postexercise electrocardiogram. Br Heart J 38:1299–1303, 1976
33. Berman DS, Salel AF, Denardo GL, Mason DT: Noninvasive detection of regional myocardial ischemia using rubidium 81 and the scintillation camera. Comparison with stress electrocardiography in patients with arteriographically documented coronary stenosis. Circulation 52:619–625, 1975
34. Strauss HW, Harrison K, Langan JK, et al: Thallium 201 for myocardial imaging. Relation of thallium 201 to regional myocardial perfusion. Circulation 51:641–647, 1975
35. Bailey IK, Griffith LSC, Rouleau J et al: Thallium-201 myocardial perfusion imaging at rest and during exercise. Comparative sensitivity to electrocardiography in coronary artery disease. Circulation 55:79–87, 1977
36. Watanabe K, Bhargava V, Froelicher V: Computer analysis of the exercise ECG: a review. Prog Cardiovasc Dis 22:423–446, 1980
37. Goldschlager N, Cake D, Cohn K: Exercise-induced ventricular arrhythmias in patients with coronary artery disease. Their relationship to angiographic findings. Am J Cardiol 31:434–440, 1973
38. McHenry PL, Morris SN, Kavalier M, Jordan JW: Comparative study of exercise-induced ventricular arrhythmias in normal subjects and patients with documented coronary artery disease. Am J Cardiol 37:609–614, 1976
39. Zaret BL, Conti CR Jr: Exercise-induced ventricular irritability: hemodynamic and angiographic correlations. Am J Cardiol 29:298–303, 1972
40. Jelinek MV, Lown B: Exercise stress testing for exposure of cardiac arrhythmias. Prog Cardiovasc Dis 16:497–522, 1974
41. Bruce RA, Kusumi F, Hosmer D: Maximal oxygen intake and nomographic assessment of functional aerobic impairment in cardiovascular disease. Am Heart J 85:546–562, 1973
42. Scheuer J, Greenberg MA, Zohman LR: Exercise training in patients with coronary artery disease. Mod Concepts Cardiovasc Dis 47:85–90, 1978

43. Gey GO, Levy RH, Fisher L, et al: Plasma concentration of procainamide and prevalence of exertional arrhythmias. Ann Intern Med 80:718–722, 1974
44. Gey GO, Levy RH, Pettet G, Fisher L: Quinidine plasma concentration and exertional arrhythmia. Am Heart J 90:19–24, 1975
45. Clausen JP, Trap-Jensen J: Heart rate and arterial blood pressure during exercise in patients with angina pectoris. Effects of training and nitroglycerin. Circulation 53:436–442, 1976
46. Bruce RA, Kusumi F, Frederick R: Differences in cardiac function with prolonged physical training for cardiac rehabilitation. Am J Cardiol 40:597–603, 1977
47. Niederberger M, Bruce RA, Kusumi F, Whitkanack S: Disparities in ventilatory and circulatory responses to bicycle and treadmill exercise. Br Heart J 36:377–382, 1974
48. Chaitman BR, Bourassa MG, Wagniart P, et al: Improved efficiency of treadmill exercise testing using a multiple lead ECG system and basic hemodynamic exercise response. Circulation 57:71–79, 1978
49. Froelicher VF Jr, Wolthius R, Keiser N, et al: A comparison of two bipolar exercise electrocardiographic leads to lead V_5. Chest 70:611–616, 1976
50. Morris SN, Phillips JF, Jordan JW, McHenry PL: Incidence and significance of decreases in systolic blood pressure during graded treadmill exercise testing. Am J Cardiol 41:221–226, 1978
51. Rochmis P, Blackburn H: Exercise tests: a survey of procedures, safety, and litigation experience in approximately 170,000 tests. JAMA 217:1061–1066, 1971

7 | Rehabilitation During the Acute and Convalescent Stages Following Myocardial Infarction

Robin S. Graf

OUTMODED CONCEPTS OF CARDIAC PATIENT CARE

Slow but dramatic progress has been made in the area of mobilizing the cardiac patient following an acute incident.[1-3] At the onset of the twentieth century, patients were forced to remain in bed for 6 to 8 weeks; they were totally at the mercy of hospital staff for even minimal self care. When hospital discharge was finally permitted, continued bedrest with strictly limited activity for an additional 3 to 6 months was common. The patient who returned to gainful employment or an otherwise productive lifestyle was the exception.

These rigid activity limitations had their base in fear, fear that any degree of physical exertion might increase hypoxemia, resulting in life threatening arrhythmias; might cause extension of the myocardial infarction, multiply the chances of ventricular aneurysm or cardiac rupture, or for other reasons result in sudden cardiac death. These fears were magnified during the initial 6 to 8 weeks post-infarction, when necrotic myocardium is converted to scar tissue.[4-7]

Early physicians and cardiologists as late as the 1970's gave only secondary importance to principles identified in the 1940's by Levine, Dock, and Harrison.[8-11] The rationale for Samuel Levine's chair treatment was based on his finding that sitting increases venous pooling, and decreases venous return and cardiac work.[10] Levine and Lown demonstrated that cardiac output was actually reduced by 23 percent when patients immediately post-infarction moved from lying supine to sitting erect in a chair.[12, 13] Similarly, De Busk found no significant increases in cardiac output or ventricular arrhythmias with postural changes or selected low level active exercises.[14] The increase in the incidence of thromboembolism with prolonged bedrest was also identified.[8]

ILL EFFECTS OF PROLONGED BEDREST

This increased chance of thromboembolism goes hand in hand with several other ill effects of bedrest. Prolonged bedrest results in hypovolemia, with the circulating blood volume decreasing 700 to 800 cc in 7 to 10 days. This hypovolemia helps to explain the moderate tachycardia and orthostatic hypotension seen after an extended period of time in the recumbent position. These changes are of particular concern for patients with a compromised myocardium. Faredduddin and Abelman concluded that this imparied orthostatic tolerance is preventable or reversible by modified bedrest or early ambulation.[15] As this hypovolemia occurs, the plasma volume decreases to a greater extent than does the red blood cell mass, resulting in increased viscosity and the above mentioned risk of thromboembolism.[16]

The aerospace program has also provided us with research on the results of prolonged immobilization.[17] The documented 20 to 25 percent decrease in maximal oxygen uptake following 21 days of strict bedrest is extremely important. At least 3 weeks of vigorous training were required to restore the pre-bedrest level of conditioning.[18] This finding goes a long way in explaining the post-illness fatigue and weakness we see in our patients, some of whom were deconditioned prior to hospital admission.

Bedrest and inactivity also cause muscle atrophy, which is accompanied by a negative nitrogen and protein balance.[16] After 1 week of bedrest the patient has experienced a 10 to 15 percent decrease in muscle contractile strength. This loss of strength causes an increase in blood pressure and myocardial oxygen consumption responses to given submaximal muscle tension levels. This adds stress to an already impaired oxygen transport system and damaged myocardium.[16]

The psychological effects of having a myocardial infarction and subsequently being confined to bedrest can be as damaging as the physical effects. Studies of the physiologic response to fear and anxiety were done by Stead in the 1940's.[19] They demonstrated that these factors markedly increase cardiac output. It was hypothesized that the concern and anxiety about invalidism and prolonged disability or death brought about by prolonged immobility might in fact increase cardiac work. The current theory is that a gradual progressive increase in activity provides visible evidence of improvement and decreases fear and anxiety.[20]

With the adverse effects of prolonged bedrest now proven and with more current research[21-23] which indicates that the fear of aneurysm formation or extension of the myocardial infarction is unjustified, early mobilization programs have been developed. Initial data from these programs confirmed that the majority of patients with uncomplicated myocardial infarctions, as evidenced by their first few days of hospitalization, have little or no in-hospital mortality and very few significant late complications.[23, 24] This information has encouraged continued early mobilization and subsequent early hospital discharge for properly selected patients.[25-27]

MODERN CARDIAC REHABILITATION PROGRAMS

The physical, psychosocial, and educational components of a comprehensive cardiac rehabilitation program should be designed and modified to meet the patient's specific and individual needs during each stage of recovery.

Early In-hospital Treatment

The first phase in the patient's recovery is his in-hospital stay. The goals here are to maintain the patient's prior level of fitness and to prevent the adverse effects of immobilization as discussed above, as well as to minimize the psychologically depressing and anxiety provoking effects of sustaining a "Heart Attack." Patient education begins immediately and is ongoing with an effort to begin changes in behavior patterns to reduce cardiovascular risk factors. The composite effect of a comprehensive program is to decrease the length of the patient's hospital stay and to launch him on the road back to a productive life.[16]

The patient's rehabilitative activities are set in motion by an order from his primary physician. This physician remains in control of the patient throughout the rehabilitation process. The team may include many skilled professionals— nurse, physical therapist, occupational therapist, social worker, dietician, and vocational rehabilitation counselor—or, in a small, more limited setting, may consist of just a medical director and one skilled professional responsible for carrying out the program.

Any patient who has sustained a myocardial infarction, has had a permanent pacemaker inserted, has been admitted for unstable angina now stabilized by medical means, or has congestive heart failure or cardiomyopathy is a potential candidate for the cardiac rehabilitation program. Some programs have adapted their treatment goals, vital sign guidelines for activity, and educational components to deal with a large congestive heart failure or cardiomyopathy population.

Following the receipt of a physician's order, the team members involved in the cardiac rehabilitation program evaluate and assess the prospective patient for candidacy and level of function. Baseline requirements for inclusion are: (1) stable vital signs, (2) absence of continued ischemia, left ventricular failure, serious circulatory impairment, important dysrhythmia, conduction defects, severe pleurisy, pericarditis, or important dysfunction of other organ systems, (3) adequate motivation by the patient to work towards the program goals, (4) significant rehabilitation potential, (5) necessity for a relatively intense, coordinated, multidisciplinary rehabilitation program, and (6) capacity of the patient or a close associate to understand the material presented and to participate meaningfully in and cooperate with the rehabilitation program. Through the pre-activity assessment discussed in Chapter 4, it is determined whether the prospective candidate has experienced a complicated (large infarction, congestive heart failure, uncontrolled dysrhythmia, shock, or intractable angina) or uncomplicated post-infarction course. This determination will affect the patient from his first treatment throughout his rehabilitative course. For the patient who has sustained an uncomplicated myocardial infarction, low level active exercise, breathing exercises, low level self care, and minimal ambulation can usually be started in the coronary care unit.[29–31] The patient's activity is monitored by a nurse or qualified therapist (Fig. 7-1). The parameters monitored are heart rate, blood pressure, electrocardiogram, and symptoms. Options for activities, as well as instructions and procedures for carrying them out, have frequently been detailed.[14, 32–34]

Indications of an inappropriately high level of activity at this stage include: an unusual heart rate increase (greater than 20 beats per minute over baseline); a systolic blood pressure increase greater than 40 mm Hg or a decrease greater than 20 mm Hg with activity (therapist will allow for orthostatic changes); diastolic blood pressure increase to greater than 110 mm Hg or a decrease greater than 15 mm Hg; and symptoms including angina, sharply increasing dyspnea, excessive fatigue, increasing mental confusion or dizziness, severe leg claudication, electrocardiogram abnormalities (including development of ischemic ST changes, serious arrhythmias, second or third degree AV block), signs of pallor, cyanosis, cold sweat, ataxia, new ventricular gallop, new regurgitation murmur, or marked increase in pulmonary rales.

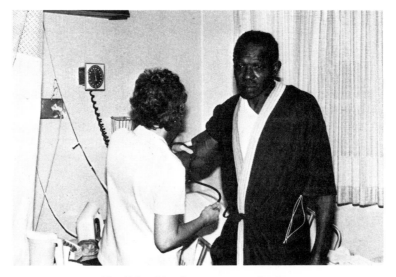

Fig. 7-1. Blood pressure monitoring.

Those patients who exhibit the above signs or symptoms or exceed the stated vital sign guidelines during activity should be withheld from treatment until the patient's primary physician has evaluated the patient's cardiac condition and the team has formulated a revised activity plan.

Later In-hospital Treatment

During the latter portion of the patient's hospital stay, the above guidelines remain in effect with a little more flexibility, including a 30 beat per minute increase in heart rate, being permitted (also see Ch. 2 for guidelines concerning exercise intensity). The above indications for terminating exercise, or those established by each individual rehabilitation team, should be adhered to unless the patient's primary physician provides specific alternate vital sign and symptom guidelines. Appropriate activities for the later portions of the patient's hospital stay include longer periods sitting in a chair, more aggressive rhythmic arm and leg exercise, and progressively longer periods of ambulation leading up to stair climbing. Many programs utilize graded calisthenic exercises to aid in the maintenance of strength and endurance of the trunk and upper extremities (see Chs. 2 and 9). Heart rate, blood pressure, electrocardiogram, and symptom monitoring continue as in the coronary care unit (Fig. 7-2). Activity sessions normally occur twice daily and last from 15 to 25 minutes as tolerated by the patient. Unnecessary isometric exercise, particularly in conjunction with a valsalva maneuver, should be avoided, to minimize chances for sudden large increases in blood pressure. Scheduling of the patient's education and activity must be done to provide a well balanced program with regards to both patient and staff time. Exercise should be withheld for 1 hour after meals. The patients are taught to monitor their response

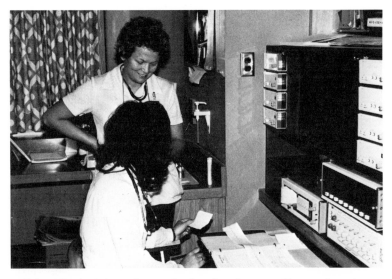

Fig. 7-2. Physical therapist monitoring the electrocardiogram by telemetry.

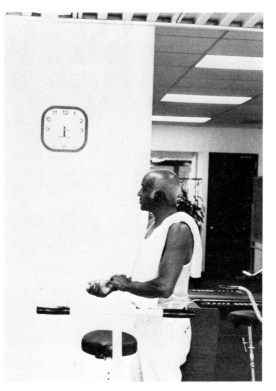

Fig. 7-3.   Patient monitoring his own pulse rate.

to activities by taking their own heart rate and becoming aware of symptoms (Fig. 7-3). If not directly supervised by a therapist in the latter phases of their hospitalization, patients may report more vigorous activities to nursing. Progress through the cardiac rehabilitation program should be as tolerated by the patient unless specific functional limitations are given by the physician.

Education and Testing

Education is provided to patients and families in coordination with the activity program. All of the involved disciplines contribute to the educational aspect of the program. This component includes the anatomy and physiology of the heart and heart attack, the healing process, symptom recognition, stages in recovery, risk factors, the effects of exercise, pacing of activities, energy conservation, dietary considerations, sexual activity, handling stress, medications, and first hour care. Those aspects not thoroughly covered on an inpatient basis should be covered during the outpatient education component.

Prior to discharge the patient will be evaluated and will receive instructions in recommended home activity level (Fig. 7-4), precautions, warning signals, and medications, and in how to contact the hospital for questions and post-hospital

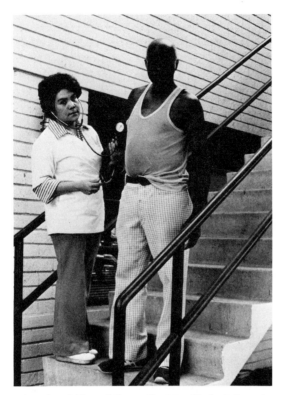

Fig. 7-4. Assessing the ability of the patient to climb stairs prior to discharge.

followup. The rehabilitation process is emphasized as a continuing lifelong process.

The low level exercise test is a very beneficial tool to the therapist attempting to assign a home program or establish an initial outpatient exercise prescription. The purpose of the test is to identify arrhythmias at low to moderate levels of activity (known exercise intensity levels); to detect abnormal ventricular function (i.e., S3, rales) with activity, abnormal blood pressure response, symptoms associated with low to moderate levels of exercise (angina, dyspnea, claudication, fatigue, dizziness); to identify bradycardic patients; and to evaluate candidacy for an outpatient exercise program.[7]

Various protocols are used in performing low level exercise testing, but many of the criteria for terminating a test are similar. These include completion of all of the protocol stages, achievement of a heart rate of 130 or more beats per minute, falling systolic blood pressure response greater than 20 mm Hg, coupled PVC's or ventricular tachycardia, more than 8 to 10 PVC's per minute, onset of angina, and a markedly hypertensive blood pressure response.

When performed by skilled personnel on appropriately selected patients using the above or similar guidelines, the low level exercise test has proven to be both safe and effective. The treadmill (Fig. 7-5) is usually the preferred ergometer

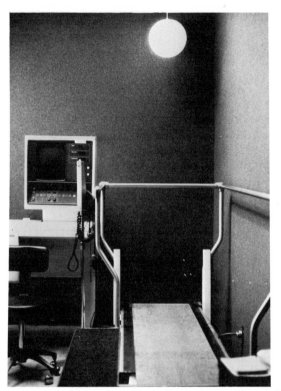

Fig. 7-5. The treadmill is used regularly for patient testing and training.

for testing. A "Crash Cart" or "Code Cart" should be available in the physical therapy department (Fig. 7-6). Besides assisting in identifying appropriate outpatient candidates, and providing them with maximum heart rate and exercise intensity guidelines for the initial phase of their out of hospital rehabilitation, it also helps in identifying patients with severe disease and the potential for future complications.

CONCLUSION

Though progress was initially slow, and despite the continuing existence of skeptical physicians, early mobilization has now established itself as an integral part of the comprehensive care of the cardiac patient. With proper patient screening and evaluation, this process of early mobilization can be safe as well as beneficial.[23–25, 29] Though there is still no conclusive evidence as to whether activity after myocardial infarction has an effect on subsequent cardiovascular morbidity or mortality, there is little doubt that selected patients have benefited from early appropriate increases in activity. These benefits include avoiding or minimizing both the effects of bedrest deconditioning and the anxiety and depression often

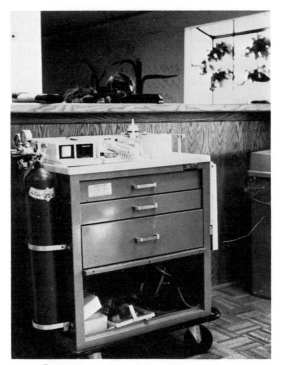

Fig. 7-6. "Crash" or "Code" Cart.

associated with having had a myocardial infarction,[20] and demonstrating an improvement rather than a decrease in physical work capacity.[36] In addition, the patient who is able to absorb and incorporate much of the program's activity and educational components is likely to put the pieces of his life back together and return to productivity more rapidly. Along with hastening the return to work, early mobilization has proven economical in decreasing the length of the patient's hospital stay.

REFERENCES

1. Duke M: Bedrest in acute myocardial infarction. A study in physician practices. Am Heart J 82:486, 1971
2. Rose G: Early mobilization and discharge after myocardial infarction. Mod Concepts Cardiovasc Dis 41:59, 1972
3. Levine SA: The myth of strict bedrest in the treatment of heart disease. Am Heart J 42:406–413, 1951
4. Jetter WW, White PD: Rupture of the heart of patients in mental institutions. Ann Intern Med 21:783, 1944
5. Mallory G, White PD, Salcedo-Salgar J: The speed of healing of myocardial infarction: a study of the pathologic anatomy in 72 cases. Am Heart J 18:647, 1939

6. Goldschlager N, Cake D, Cohn K: Exercise-induced ventricular arrhythmias in patients with coronary artery disease. Am J Cardiol 31:434–440, 1973

7. Ericsson M, Granath A, Ohlsen P, et al: Arrhythmias and symptoms during treadmill testing 3 weeks after myocardial infarction in 100 patients. Br Heart J 35:787–790, 1973

8. Dock W: The evil sequelae of complete bedrest. JAMA 125:1083, 1944

9. Harrison TR: Abuse of rest as a therapeutic measure for patients with cardiovascular disease. JAMA 125:1075, 1944

10. Levine SA, Lown B: The "chair" treatment of acute coronary thrombosis. Trans Assoc Am Physicians 64:316, 1951

11. Irvin CW, Burgess AM: The abuse of bedrest in the treatment of myocardial infarction. N Engl J Med 283:486–489, 1950

12. Levine SA, Lown B: Armchair treatment of acute coronary thrombosis. JAMA 148:1365–1369, 1952

13. Coe WS: Cardiac work and the chair treatment of coronary thrombosis. Ann Intern Med 40:42–48, 1954

14. Debusk RF, Spivak AP, VanKessel A, et al: The coronary care units activity program: its role in post-infarction rehabilitation. J Chronic Dis 24:373–381, 1971

15. Faredduddin K, Abelman WH: Impaired orthostatic tolerance in patients with myocardial infarction. N Engl J Med 280:345–350, 1969

16. Wenger NK: Exercise and the Heart. Philadelphia, FA Davis, 1978

17. Miller PB, Johnson RL, Lamb LE: Effects of moderate physical exercise during 4 weeks of bedrest on the circulatory function of man. Aerosp Med 36:1077–1078, 1965

18. Saltin B, Blomquist G, Mitchell JH: Response to exercise after bedrest and training. Circulation 37–38 (suppl 7):1, 1968

19. Stead EA Jr, Warren JV, Merrill AJ: The cardiac output in male subjects as measured by the technique of right atrial catheterization, normal values with observations of the effects of anxiety and tilting. J Clin Invest 24:326, 1944

20. McPherson BD, Palvio A, Yuhasz MS: Psychological effects of an exercise program on post-infarction and normal adult men. J Sports Med Phys Fitness 7:95–102, 1967

21. Thomas WC, Harrison TR: The effects of artificial restriction of activity on the recovery of rats from experimental myocardial injury. Am J Med Sci 208:436–450, 1944

22. Kaplinsky E, Hood WB, McCarthy B: Effects of physical training in dogs with coronary artery ligation. Circulation 37:356–365, 1968

23. Thompson PL, Jenzer HR, Lown B, et al: Exercise during acute myocardial infarction: an experimental study. Cardiovasc Res 7:642–648, 1973

24. Boyle JA, Lorimer AR, Douglas AS: Early mobilization after acute myocardial infarction. prospective study of 338 patients. Lancet 2:346, 1973

25. Harpur JE, Kellett RJ, Conner WT: Controlled trial of early mobilization in uncomplicated myocardial infarction. Lancet 2:1331, 1971

26. Hutter AM, Sidel VW, Shine KL: Early hospital discharge after myocardial infarction. N Engl J Med 228:142, 1973

27. Swan HJC, Blackburn HW, DeSanctis R: Duration of hospitalization in "uncomplicated completed myocardial infarction." An ad hoc committee review. Am J Cardiol 37:413, 1976

28. California Hospital Medical Center Inpatient Cardiac Rehabilitation Protocol. Los Angeles, CA, revised July, 1980

29. Lamers HJ, Drast WSJ, Kroon BJM: Early mobilization after a myocardial infarction: a controlled study. Br J Med 1:257, 1973

30. Bloch A, Maeder JP, Haissley JC: Early mobilization after a myocardial infarction: a controlled study. Am J Cardiol 34: 152, 1974

31. Groden BM: The management of myocardial infarction. A controlled study of the effects of early mobilization. Cardiac Rehabil 1:13, 1971
32. Myocardial Infarction: How to Prevent, How to Rehabilitate. Council on Rehabilitation, International Society of Cardiology: 1973
33. Wenger NK: Cardiac inpatient conditioning program (Appendix 4). J SC Med Assoc 65 (suppl 8):102–104, 1969
34. Cardiac Rehabilitation 1975. Report of a joint working party of the Royal College of Physicians of London and the British Society on Rehabilitation after Cardiac Illness. J R Coll Physicians Lond 9:281–346, 1975
35. Guidelines for Cardiac Rehabilitation Centers. The American Heart Association Greater Los Angeles Affiliate, Cardiac Rehabilitation Committee, Los Angeles, 1978
36. Detry JM: Exercise Testing and Training in Coronary Heart Disease. Baltimore, Williams & Wilkins, 1973

8 | Cardiac Rehabilitation of Outpatients During the Recovery Stage Following Myocardial Infarction

Charles L. Carter

Exercise intervention in chronic disease is well known to the physical therapist. Outpatient cardiac rehabilitation (OCR) has become a logical extension of the physical therapy clinic. Outpatient care is the final expression of the goals in the team approach to cardiac rehabilitation. OCR can offer lasting physiological and psychological benefit to the post-myocardial infarction (Post-MI) patient. The program will eventually remove the dependence of medical personnel, and promote individual habits which serve to maintain exercise training and reduce risk factors.

The basic components of outpatient rehabilitation are: the patient referral process, the exercise prescription, the basic program design, and the safe supervision of this high risk patient. The patient will in most cases progress smoothly to the final outpatient discharge and subsequent independence, if these components are properly "fit" to the patient.

SELECTION OF THE PATIENT

A simple listing of the contraindications to exercise may be helpful in screening patients for the program (Table 8-1). A complete listing of contraindications to exercise and exercise testing is available.[1, 2] Acute illness, uncontrolled chronic systemic disease, uncontrolled arrhythmia, unstable angina, severe aortic stenosis, and basically any highly unstable disease process are logically excluded from the program. The literature provides very little data to support the description of the best screening procedure. It is clear, however, that screening must include a complete history, a complete physical, and a graded exercise test (GXT).[3] The ultimate goal of the evaluation is to enable the physician to make accurate clinical judgments by providing him with the best quantitative information possible.

Keep in mind that a graded exercise test may be indicated to provide important functional information, even though chronic exercise may not be sound treatment. The value of exercise training for hypertensive patients with diastolic pressure greater than 120 mm Hg is controversial.[3, 4] It is important for the therapist to review the chart with special attention to the type and severity of myocardial infarction and to the medication record. It is also important to interview the potential patient just prior to his scheduled GXT, to identify symptoms. At this time, you determine the stability of the anginal pattern. The needed information is sometimes hard to elicit. Ask these questions (1) does chest pain occur without exercise or other provocation? (2) is the pain more intense or frequent when last noted, compared to previous episodes (crescendo angina)? (3) does it last longer than 3 to 5 minutes? An affirmative answer to these simple inquiries suggests the possibility of unstable angina or preinfarction syndrome and the GXT, let alone outpatient rehabilitation, is contraindicated.

A thorough chest wall exam is indicated, utilizing motion to help identify pain of musculo-skeletal origin. After the application of the multiple ECG leads, auscultate the chest with the bell of the stethoscope at an accessible intercostal space (e.g., left sternal border third intercostal space) for the presence or absence of a third or fourth heart sound at rest and after exercise. This will assist in the determination of the presence or absence of left ventricular impairment. While these simple procedures may at first seem unimportant, familiarity with the patient's signs and symptoms, his medical history, and his response to graded exercise are vital to physical therapy management of that patient. For a more complete review of patient assessment see Part II.

Table 8-1. Medical Findings That Contraindicate Exercise Training[3-6]

Acute myocardial infarction	Bilateral bundle branch block
Unstable angina or impending infarction	Type II second degree AV block
Overt symptoms of congestive heart failure	Complete heart block
Severe three vessel coronary artery stenosis	Uncontrolled diabetes
Dangerous uncontrolled arrhythmia	Myocarditis
Exercise induced arrhythmia (untreated)	Acute thrombophlebitis
Large ventricular aneurysms	Overt psychosis
Advanced aortic stenosis	

Determine the patient's approximate lean body mass by either underwater weighing or with skin fold calipers and tape measure. It is important for positive feedback and patient self-image to learn of his loss of fat or replacement of fat with muscle. Often a patient's body weight will not change significantly, and if lean body mass has not been measured, this could lead to a loss of interest in the program.

The total money available for cardiac rehabilitation does have limits. Therefore, it is important that the initial screening determine both the patient's own goals and his motivation for cardiac rehabilitation. This is a good chance for the therapist and the patient to exchange expectations. Most often, patients who are financially rewarded for disability or those who express a very negative attitude toward exercise do not adhere to the program.[3]

If a risk factor assessment has been completed, add this information to the outpatient records. If an assessment has not been completed, gather the following information: (1) age, (2) sex, (3) B.P. (hypertension?), (4) serum cholesterol and high density alpha lipoproteins, if possible, (5) cigarette smoker, (6) previous and present level of activity, (7) forced vital capacity, (8) family history of coronary artery disease, and (9) diabetes mellitus. Informed consent also needs to be obtained. For an excellent form see page 53 of *Exercise Testing and Training of Individuals with Heart Disease or at High Risk for Its Development: A Handbook for Physicians,* published in 1975 by the Committee on Exercise of the American Heart Association.

For angina patients it is also important to determine the daily intake of xanthines (caffeine) and other stimulants that often elevate resting heart rate and are responsible for increased daily angina. While caffeine has not been studied as a risk factor, reduction of caffeine intake by the use of decaffeinated coffee may reduce anginal complaints in a number of patients.

EXERCISE PRESCRIPTION

The central focus of an outpatient program is an accurate graded exercise testing facility. The information gathered from these tests, together with the patient interview, allow the generation of an exercise prescription. Chronic exercise will, in most cases, elicit potent changes that are often as intense as those elicited by prescription medications. It is, therefore, important to specify intensity, duration, and frequency, as well as mode of exercise.[1]

Intensity

An exercise prescription for symptomatic post-MI patients must have a safety buffer zone built into it. Patients that have a symptom limited maximal capacity (SL_{max}) deserve special care in the writing of an exercise prescription.

There are two reasonable approaches to selecting a range. You should be consistent in your program and use the same formula throughout. The simpler procedure, which has been recommended by the Committee on Exercise in *Exer-*

cise Testing and Training of Apparently Healthy Individuals: A Handbook for Physicians published in 1972 by the American Heart Association, is to use a target heart rate of 70 to 85 percent of the maximum attainable heart rate achieved during the GXT. Thus, this group recommends a training range or "target zone" to bring about an effective training response. There is continuous controversy regarding the lowest intensity level required to give a training response. It does appear that a load should elicit greater than 50 percent of the patient's maximal capacity.[7]

The second procedure to determine intensity is to determine the working heart range by the following formula:[8]

$$HR_{\text{working range}} = (HR_{\text{maximum achieved}}) - (HR_{\text{rest}})$$

Then determine 60 percent of the range, and add this to the resting heart rate.

$$HR_{\text{target}} = (60 \text{ percent} \times HR_{\text{working range}}) + (HR_{\text{rest}})$$

While this procedure is slightly more complicated, it does yield a specific target intensity. One should not assume, however, that this specific target heart rate can be strictly adhered to for an entire 15 to 20 min training period. Also, since the resting heart rate will diminish with training and the reduction in caffeine intake, the precise target heart rate may be difficult to calculate.

If you are starting a new program from scratch, you may appreciate the flexibility of using 70 to 85 percent of maximum heart rate as the target zone. This is usually a conservative intensity and does not involve the problem of measuring an accurate resting heart rate before a GXT.

Duration and Frequency

Duration and frequency in the rehabilitation program are important, because treatment time, as with any therapeutic procedure, should be directed at the optimal cost benefit to the patient. There is evidence to support an optimal duration of 20 minutes per day, and 3 day per week frequency.[7] The exercise days are to be separated by days of rest. A specific time to re-test the patient to assess his prognosis and to limit the duration of this prescription should be included.

Mode of Exercise

The mode of exercise should always be considered in the prescription. The patient response should be predictable to both the patient and the program personnel. The wise procedure is to evaluate the patient with the same exercise he will use for training. For example, if a bicycle ergometer will be used, then evaluate the patient on a bicycle ergometer. Select continuous movement exercises that involve large muscle mass, and thereby avoid unpredictable reflexes such as the valsalva.

Program Design

The key considerations in program design are safe, noncompetitive activities, goal directed for each patient. Emphasize improvement in self-concept by stressing knowledge of results and individual responsibility for altering risk factors. Relaxation technique should be part of every program as well, to arm the patient with specific tools to deal with job and home related stresses. You should share your knowledge of exercise physiology with your patients. A number of patients will even respond to a presentation of your new findings in the literature as they relate to exercise and the heart. Your best patients will usually be the best informed patients as well. The fact that your patients are taking part in a treatment (which they literally give to themselves under supervision) in which all ramifications and questions will not be answered for perhaps 20 to 30 years may actually stimulate them to adhere to the prescription. They are actually adding to an understanding of the value of exercise as a therapeutic agent. Cardiac patients are often very interested in understanding their disease, so a routine educational program will improve interest and encourage adherence.

Even though your most enthusiastic patients may be very competitive individuals, it is important continuously to discourage competition between patients. Design each session with a timed warm-up period, a walk or jog to target period, and a definite cool down period. Monitor each patient's radial pulse before he leaves the exercise session to assure that he is not adversely responding to the activity. Suggested low level activities during the warm-up period are group interaction games with a ball; for example, volleyball where the ball is permitted one bounce before it is returned to the opposite side. Other reasonable warm-up activities are graded calisthenics,[10] walking sequences, or moderate stretching and joint mobilization exercises. Avoid sit-ups in most cases, because heart rate responses are often unpredictable.[5] Design each session with the individual patient in mind. There will be some patients who do not choose group treatment sessions. If the patients do not know their responses well or have not learned how to monitor themselves accurately, insist that they attend supervised sessions until they are independent in self-monitoring. The unsupervised exercise prescription should consist of exercises of lower intensity and longer duration to provide a greater than 15 beat buffer zone from the symptomatic heart rate. Low level activities such as slower walking are greatly preferred for the unsupervised post-MI patient. Drop the target heart rate down at least 5 to 10 beats and walk with the patient until he knows the ambulatory rate which will achieve that target and is able to monitor himself.

When you select activities, keep in mind the way the heart "sees" the activity. Cardiac patients and unfit patients require significantly more coronary blood flow per 100 g of myocardium than normal individuals while working at approximately the same workload.[5] This is especially true of patients with moderate to large infarcts who have akinetic or dyskinetic segments of the heart. Therefore, a patient with an akinetic heart wall who performs an exercise, side by side, at the same cadence and workload as another post-MI patient with a healed sub-endocardinal infarct, may be far exceeding his ischemic threshold. There will be a lag between the onset of the exercise, and heart response. There will also be a period when the activity seems well tolerated when in fact it is not.

Individual goals should be established for each patient, which could include the following:

1. Returning to work
2. Improved submaximal and maximal performance
3. Lower HR and SBP at the same submaximal workload
4. Reduced exercise induced extrasystoles
5. Improved sexual performance
6. Decreased total body fat
7. Reduced occurrence of angina per day
8. Stopping smoking
9. Improved stress tolerance
10. Reduced depression
11. Better "quality of life"

Note that the first eight goals may be quantitatively measured. It is exceedingly important to make appropriate measurements, to determine specific progress to reinforce the hard effort the patient is putting forth. You can expect progress toward many of these goals by the vast majority of your patients.[11]

The final program design component is instruction and practice in relaxation technique. Selye has recommended that we either physically remove ourselves from stress, or learn to relax, in order to prevent general stress reactions.[12] Perhaps a major reason why your patient is in a cardiac rehabilitation program is that mounting tension has not been followed by action. This condition constitutes an accelerating stress to that individual. The myocardial infarction is, in most cases, a stress release. Without a knowledge of how to recognize and deal with this tension, complex feelings of guilt, self-doubt, and low self esteem may be amplified. Your patients under 50 may be as much as 5 times more anxious than a healthy control group.[13]

Jacobson techniques of progressive relaxation of body regions are effective with post-MI patients.[14] Monographs are available that describe effective relaxation exercises in detail.[15] There is controversy regarding the permanent benefits that accompany this kind of training in post-MI patients. However, knowledge of how to sense and subsequently release chronically tight musculature during any stressful period will be an effective tool to build confidence and self-concept. Many patients relate life's stresses to their heart disease. Therefore, any procedure that gives them confidence in handling these stresses will reduce anxiety. These sessions are most effectively taught in a quiet private area. Practice sessions may be monitored by a properly trained aide. Once the patient has mastered the techniques, you may reinforce his success by noting his heart rate and blood pressure before and after a session. Work on specific techniques that may be continued on-the-job as well as at home. At least one relaxation session with the spouse is mandatory.

SUPERVISION OF THE PATIENT AND PRECAUTIONS

All outpatient post-MI programs must have a shock cart with a DC defibrillator at the site of activity. An ECG capable of monitoring the CM5 lead configuration is also necessary. A good clock that all can see, and a telephone are also basic necessities. There should be a staff member, certified in the use of equipment, present at the site during all periods of activity as well. The American Heart Association has made it clear that *direct* physician supervision of testing and training, while desirable, is "not always necessary," when the staff are trained in CPR and emergency cardiac care.[1, 2]

Other desirable monitoring equipment is at least one ECG telemetry unit and access to a Holter monitor. The telemetry is very useful for accurate determination of the exercise intensity during upper extremity work, when radial pulse monitoring is difficult, if not impossible. The real value of telemetry, however, is the detection of exercise induced arrhythmia. When patients complain of skipped beats during certain kinds of work activity, reproduce that activity while they are monitored. If the arrhythmia cannot be uncovered in this manner, 24-hour monitoring with a tape recorder is preferable. Paroxysmal atrial tachycardia (PAT) is best studied with the 24-hour Holter monitor, as are other arhythmias that cannot be induced in an exercise testing or training session. This close monitoring as well as your clinical observation will greatly assist in the determination of the safest level of antiarrhythmia agents. Your patient will often walk the fine line between the dose needed to suppress the arrhythmia and severe diarrhea or other symptom of drug intolerance. Your job is to help "fine tune" the dosage.

Major supervisory problems may be lessened by an outline of the duration of all activities. This scheduling can effectively reduce the number of unknowns you can expect to see at the training session, thus making the program predictable from session to session. Schedule routine monitoring of the radial pulse on each patient during the peak of all activities. Monitoring is especially mandatory on all new activities. Finally, it is best to walk or jog to target heart rate on a one to one basis until your new patient becomes familiar with his own monitoring, as well as with the limits of his exercise prescription. You will find that post-MI patient supervision is not, in principle, different from what you are accustomed to.

RE-EVALUATION OF THE PATIENT

As in all forms of therapy, re-evaluation of the patient is very important. Retest the patient on the identical exercise GXT protocol as he completed for the exercise prescription. The purpose of the repeat GXT is to provide feedback to the patient as well as to determine how much training has taken place. Stated otherwise, are the goals being achieved? It is a time in which medications need to be re-evaluated. Remember that exercise prescriptions written while the patient was on certain medications (e.g. propranolol) are not valid after a significant change in medications.

It is suggested that you draw a "work diagram" for each patient. Plot the heart rate (y-axis) versus the work load and the double product (SBP $\times$ HR $\times 10^{-3}$) versus the work load on the same sheet of paper. Use thin enough paper to allow you to superimpose each repeat GXT, to demonstrate visually to the patient his increase/decrease in capacity and heart rate at each exercise intensity. This is a comfortable tool for reflecting on the goals that have been set. Draw in the anginal threshold or point where symptoms occurred.

During the re-evaluation period, note any changes that have been made in risk factors, specific changes in anginal threshold (work level and double product), and how much nitroglycerin is required during a week and why. Re-estimate lean body mass by the formula that best fits your population of patients. Finally, determine qualitatively whether your patient is gaining a better life (sex, available energy, better self-image) from his effort.

RECORD KEEPING

There are a number of reasons for keeping good records in addition to the legal requirements for documentation. Recognize that your population of patients is unique and can contribute to our understanding of cardiac rehabilitation. Furthermore, you will learn more about what to expect from patients over the 1 to 5 year period of expected observation.

Document daily treatment heart rates versus specific activities. The patients themselves can assist you with this record. Record on the same document the symptoms and other notable responses. Record all arrhythmias that occur or changes in pattern that can be identified. Keep in mind that you are in essence completing the coronary care unit (CCU) records so keep them available and refer back to them when you don't understand a patient response. Finally, keep records of caffeine intake, smoking, and metabolic and emotional job demands. Follow-up calls to each patient 1 year, 2 years, and at 3 to 5 years post-MI would be the best possible follow-up to complete the patient file.

FUTURE PROSPECTS

There will be a number of controversies resolved in the near future, allowing better design of the post-MI rehabilitation program. These include: (1) significance of the cardiac changes that occur with exercise, (2) the level of training necessary to alter the course of the disease, (3) psychological effects of the cause of the disease, (4) infarct size and training effects, (5) problems of de-training, (6) sudden-death syndrome, (7) diet and the course of the disease when coupled with exercise, and (8) significance of the difference between a "normal" patient response and a post-MI patient response.

This chapter was written for the purpose of facilitating your participation in cardiac rehabilitation treatment and clinical research. It is designed as only a beginning point in outpatient post-MI rehabilitation training.

REFERENCES

1. Committee on Exercise: Exercise Testing and Training of Individuals with Heart Disease or at High Risk for Its Development: A Handbook for Physicians. New York, American Heart Association, 1975
2. Fox SM, Naughton JP, Gorman PA: Modern Concepts of Cardiovascular Disease: Physical Activity and Cardiovascular Health. New York, American Heart Association, 1972
3. McHenry MM: Medical screening of patients with coronary artery disease. Am J Cardiol 33:752–755, 1974
4. Boyer JL, Kasch FW: Exercise therapy in hypertensive men. JAMA 211:1669–1671, 1970
5. Hellerstein HK, Hirsch E, Ader R, et al: Principles of exercise prescription. In: Exercise Testing and Exercise Training in Coronary Heart Disease, ed. Naughton J, Hellerstein HK. New York, Academic Press, 1973
6. Fox SM, Naughton JP, Haskell WL: Physical activity and the prevention of coronary heart disease. Ann Clin res 3:404, 1971
7. Åstrand P, Rodahl K: Textbook of Work Physiology. New York, McGraw-Hill, 1977
8. Karvonen JJ, Kentala E, Mustala O: The effects of training on heart rate. Ann Med Exp Biol Fenn 35:307, 1957
9. Pollock ML: The quantification of endurance training programs. In: Exercise and Sports Science Reviews, ed. Wilmore JH. New York, Academic Press, 1973
10. Amundsen LR, Takahashi M, Carter CL, Nielson DH: Energy cost of rehabilitation calisthenics. Phy Ther 59:855–858, 1979
11. Hellerstein HK, Hornsten TR, Goldbarg A, et al: The influence of active conditioning upon subjects with coronary artery disease. Can Med Assoc J 96:12, 1967
12. Selye H: The Stress of Life. New York, McGraw-Hill, 1956
13. Rodda BE, Miller MC, Bruhn JG: Prediction of anxiety and depression patterns among coronary patients using a Markov process analysis. Behav Sci 16:482–489, 1971
14. Jacobsen E: Progressive Relaxation. Chicago, University of Chicago Press, 1938
15. Rathbone JL: Relaxation. Philadelphia, Lea and Febiger, 1969

9 | Case Study: Rehabilitation Following a Myocardial Infarction, with a Sample Program

Kathleen Janikula Fleischaker
Mary A. Gower
Lois M. Canafax
Louise June Holt

INTRODUCTION AND HISTORY

The purpose of this chapter is to follow a patient's progression through a cardiac rehabilitation program. This case study illustrates the extent of recovery that is possible.

The subject is a 53-year-old male who suffered an acute anteroseptal MI in July 1979 and was treated in the full cardiac rehabilitation program. The patient is a well-developed, generally healthy individual with a history of type IV hyperlipidemia, elevated cholesterol (259 mg/dl), well-controlled hypertension, and chronic knee problems due to old football injuries. He had been a light smoker until 1952, when he quit, and his family history is negative for cardiac problems. He is a college professor (Doctor of Finance).

The patient had no previous history of MIs but was diagnosed with coronary artery disease in May 1977, when a stress test done while the patient was on Inderol revealed a 1 mm junctional ST segment depression. A coronary angiogram done subsequently demonstrated an 80 percent stenosis in the circumflex artery after the distal takeoff of the obtuse marginal branch, with some sclerosis of the left anterior descending and right coronary arteries that was felt at that time to be not significant. He was placed on a 1000-Cal low-fat diet and home exercise program and did not have any discomfort suggestive of angina until the events leading to his MI.

Six weeks prior to his MI the patient noticed some episodic aching across both shoulders and under the left scapula. Three weeks later this developed into anterior chest tightness occurring sometimes with exercise and resolving with continued activity and sometimes at rest. In mid-July the patient awakened two consecutive nights with tightness and mild dyspnea across the upper chest lasting 3–4 hours and unrelieved by four or five nitorglycerin tablets of questionable age. He was admitted to the hospital ER with chest pain on July 18 and placed in the critical coronary care unit for treatment of pain and evaluation of the coronary insufficiency. EKG indicated a normal sinus rhythm of 66 bpm, with rare premature ventricular complexes and a borderline first-degree block (PR interval 0.194 mm). Some ST segment depression with T wave inversion was present, indicative of changes in the left anterior descending arterial distribution. A modest elevation of the enzymes was observed although it was felt that the peak had been missed because the patient had not sought hospitalization until 24–36 hours after the prolonged episodes of pain. A diagnosis was made of an anteroseptal infarction and an uncomplicated recovery pattern was observed.

INPATIENT HOSPITAL STAY

The patient tolerated his 3-day stay in the critical coronary unit well, with normal sinus rhythm rates of 66–70/min, continued PR interval of 0.20 mm and no complaints of dyspnea, angina, or other complications. He was given supplemental O_2, Inderal for control of hypertension, and Valium and Tylenol as needed for pain and he was placed on a 1000-Cal low-sodium soft-food diet. Activity was kept at a minimum, with commode privileges and 45 min b.i.d. chair sitting as the only exceptions to bedrest.

On July 20 the patient was transferred to the postcoronary floor, where he remained through the duration of his hospitalization. He was initially monitored with telemetry and was continued on the same diet and medications with the addition of heparin and coumadin for antiocoagulation. He was gradually given increased activity privileges, such as walking to the bathroom and shower, and in the halls with decreased supervision. Coronary education material and periodic monitoring of activity tolerance were also provided by the nursing staff.

INPATIENT CARDIAC REHABILITATION PROGRAM

The patient was referred into the three-stage Inpatient Cardiac Rehabilitation Program 5 days after his admission. The three stages consist of progressive exercises starting at lower basal metabolism (MET) level and increasing in complexity. Initially, these exercises are performed while in bed primarily to aid blood circulation and to maintain muscle tone and flexibility. Gradual increased physical activity, including rhythmic calisthenic exercise, walking, and stair climbing, are performed during the remainder of the hospital stay. (See Appendix A for a complete description of the program.)

Stage I exercises consist of active-assistive or active range-of-motion exercises to arms and legs, deep-breathing exercise, and active ankle motion while lying in bed.

Stage II exercises consist of calisthenics—starting with 1 min and increasing to 8 min—while sitting in a chair, plus some active hip, knee, and ankle motions.

Stage III exercises consist of calisthenics—beginning at 8 min and increasing to 16 min—done while standing, and of supervised walking and stair climbing.

The physical therapy department home program consists of the same calisthenic-type exercises that are performed while in the hospital along with instruction for a gradual increase of activity and energy expenditure. There is also a structured walking program available (see Appendix A).

The patient progressed well through the series of three exercise stages. Treatment was given by a physical therapist, and patient tolerance was monitored throughout. Treatment began with b.i.d. active-assistive range-of-motion exercises done bedside. These exercises were tolerated well, with minimal pulse increase from 58 to 60 bpm. Exercises were then gradually increased to b.i.d. active calisthenics done sitting and then standing at progressively higher MET levels (1.5–3.2 METs) and time intervals (2–12 min). As the patient progressed through the stages of the program, the treatment also included supervised walking and stair climbing. The patient's resting heart rate during these stages averaged 60–64 bpm with a slight increase to 66–70 bpm following exercise. All exercise sessions were tolerated well and without symptoms.

The patient was discharged from the hospital on August 1 with prescriptions for Coumadin, Inderal, Isordil, and nitroglycerin and instructions to continue the 1000-Cal, low-sodium, low-cholesterol diet. He was provided with a home program of calisthenics at 2.3–3.2 MET levels for 12 min and was ordered to continue exercise therapy as an outpatient.

OUTPATIENT CARDIAC REHABILITATION PROGRAM

The outpatient cardiac rehabilitation program consists of cardiovascular conditioning, improvement of physical fitness and exercise tolerance, education with regard to the disease process, and development of positive psychological adjustment. Individual exercise levels are set from the results of an exercise EKG test (Naughton's protocol) performed prior to initiation of the program.

Prior to beginning the outpatient cardiac rehabilitation program, the patient was given a treadmill stress test according to Naughton's protocol. The test was stopped after 5.5 min of exercise because of complaints of upper chest pain and burning with a heart rate of 99 bpm; it was designated a positive test for myocardial ischemia. From these results the physician prescribed an initial workload of 1.5 METs with heart rate limit of 95 bpm.

The patient began the rehabilitation program in August 1979 and participated three times per week. Each exercise session consisted of 5 min of warm-up calisthenics, 28 min of exercise on bicycle ergometers (including warm-ups, full training workload, and cool-downs), and 5 min of cool-down calisthenics. Throughout the exercise the patient's heart rate, blood pressure, and EKG were monitored by an RPT and an RN, and the results were charted and reported regularly to the physician. A complete description of the outpatient cardiac rehabilitation program is given in Appendix B.

The patient began exercising at a workload of 1.5 METs, and this was gradually increased to 3.8 METs during the first week to achieve a rise in heart rate. He continued at this workload for 3 weeks while remaining asymptomatic and achieving maximum systolic blood pressure of 115–125 mm Hg, maximum heart rate of 88–92 bpm, and stable EKG rhythm with some ST segment depression and very rare single PVCs. This workload was then increased to 4.8 METs, which resulted in increased systolic blood pressure of 124–140 mm Hg, increased heart rate of 88–96 bpm, increased ST depression of 0.5–1 mm, and tightness in the substernal area of the upper back. This angina was relieved by NTG but continually occurred at this workload; thus it was decided after two sessions to decrease the workload to 3.0–3.8 METs until the patient could better tolerate exercise. (It should be noted that the combination of ST segment depression and symptoms is atypical in that most patients observed in the department remain asymptomatic although ST segment depression indicates myocardial ischemia.)

The exercise workload was maintained at 3.8 METs during the next 2½ weeks, which resulted in maximum systolic blood pressure of 120–136 mm Hg, heart rate of 80–90 bpm, essentially stable rhythm, and no symptoms. During this time one session of 4.8 METs was attempted with resulting angina, minimal ST changes, and a brief episode of bigeminal rhythm.

After 8 weeks of the program the workload was increased to 4.8 METs again, and the patient was then able to tolerate this well for three sessions with essentially stable rhythms, maximum systolic blood pressure of 130 mm Hg, and heart rate of 86–90 bpm. The workload was then increased to 5.1 METs and was maintained at this level for 4 weeks. This resulted in maximum systolic blood pressure of 118–124 mm Hg, maximum heart rate of 84–94 bpm, and stable rhythms with only rare single PVCs and minimal ST changes. Workloads of 5.6 METs were attempted twice during this time but caused slight angina and increased ST depression, and were not continued.

During this time the patient had a second angiogram performed to evaluate severity of arterial occlusion, the causes of angina, and the possibility of surgical bypass intervention. The findings demonstrated significant disease in both left vessels with mild involvement of the right and an increase in plaque formation in all three major coronary arteries in comparison to the previous study. The right coronary artery contained diffuse disease with less than 50 percent narrowing, and the left circumflex artery was now totally occluded in the midportion distal to the obtuse marginal branch; collateral circulation from the obtuse marginal to the distal branches of the left circumflex artery was noted. A diagonal branch from the left anterior descending artery was observed with a 70–80 percent stenosis in the proximal portion, and the left anterior descending artery itself was 70 percent stenosed below this branch. A ventriculogram at this time showed a mild reduction in left ventricular contractility. The ejection fraction was determined to be 76 percent, and a very faint ejection murmur was noted at the left sternal border. It was decided to postpone a decision for surgical bypass and to continue the patient on the outpatient rehabilitation program at gradually increasing workloads as he could tolerate.

The workload was increased to 5.6 METs in the 13th week of treatment and was tolerated well, with maximum systolic blood pressure of 124–130 mm Hg, heart rate of 86–90 bpm, and stable rhythms. Despite two sessions missed due to influenza, the patient was able to increase his workload to 6.1 METs in the 14th week with a maximum systolic blood pressure of 122–142 mm Hg, heart rate of 96–102 bpm, and stable rhythm.

In the 15th treatment week the workload was increased to 6.5 METs, and this was maintained for 4 weeks. On several occasions during this time the patient complained of mild anginal tightness between the scapulae; this was associated with slight ST segment depression and isolated PVCs and PACs. Lower resting heart rate of 45–55 bpm and stystolic blood pressure drops to 80 mm Hg were also noted, and Inderol dosages were then decreased to 40 mg b.i.d. Average maximum systolic blood pressure values for this workload measured 130–150 mm Hg, with average maximum heart rates of 92–106 bpm.

A workload of 7.0 METs was achieved in the 19th week and, was maintained for 2 weeks with maximum systolic blood pressure values of 142–152 mm Hg, maximum heart rate of 96–108 bpm, and asymptomatic stable rhythms with rare isolated PVCs and premature nodal contractions. In the 21st week the workload was increased to 7.5 METs and the patient tolerated this well, with systolic blood pressure of 146–166 mm Hg, heart rate of 116–124 bpm, and stable rhythms. At this time he purchased a bicycle ergometer for home use and was discharged from the formal rehabilitation program. His home program instructions included daily exercise sessions of the same design as those in the department, beginning at a 7.5 MET workload with heart rate guidelines of 100–125 bpm.

The patient reported that he had faithfully continued daily home exercises at gradually increasing workloads from his time of discharge in January, 1980. He was seen for a followup exercise session 5 months later and was exercised at his new workload of 10.1 METs. This resulted in a maximum systolic blood pressure of 142 mm Hg, maximum heart rate of 118 bpm, a stable rhythm with 0.5 mm of ST segment depression, a single PVC, and no complaints of angina symptoms. Four months after this visit the patient reported that he was exercising 6 days per week at an increased workload of 10.8 METs, intending to continue this progression as he could tolerate. The patient's goal was to attain 12.0 METs by the end of 1980.

In addition to the incredible exercise achievements of this patient, he continues to maintain his weight at a level 35–40 pounds below that prior to his MI on a low-cholesterol, low-sodium diet, remains a nonsmoker, and works full-time as a college professor.

Although the outpatient cardiac rehabilitation program has proved successful for many patients, it should be noted that the extreme gains made by this subject are atypical. The majority of MI and coronary bypass patients have been initially exercised at 3–4 MET levels and have gradually progressed to maximum levels of 6–8 METs while in the department and through home aerobic exercise programs. Several patients have had to maintain lower workload levels due to repeated bouts of pericarditis or angina; several have had to discontinue the program due to recurrent angina and have needed coronary bypass surgery.

Although few patients have the abilities and the motivation to achieve the extreme improvement made by this case subject, most have agreed that the program has been beneficial in increasing their activity levels and tolerance to exercise, knowledge of coronary information, and psychological adjustment to cardiac problems. It is hoped that programs such as this will offer the cardiac patient a safe and supportive environment in which to progress to his or her maximum rehabilitation level.

ACKNOWLEDGMENT

The authors express appreciation for the cooperation of Kamal K. Sahgal, M.D., Medical Advisor for Cardiac Rehabilitation, and Samuel E. Carlson, M.D., Attending Physician, Methodist Hospital, St. Louis Park, Minn.

Appendix A

Inpatient Cardiac Rehabilitation Program
Department of Rehabilitation Medicine
Methodist Hospital
St. Louis Park, Minn.

TABLE OF CONTENTS

A-1   An Overview of the Team Approach to Inpatient Cardiac Rehabilitation

Three-stage program: 2–3 weeks
    Coronary Care Stage (stage I)   Rehab. days 1–5
    Subacute Stage (stage II)   Rehab. days 6–10
    Convalescent stage (stage III)   Rehab. days 11–15

I. *CCU Stage* (energy exenditure of 1.0–1.5 × basal metabolism): Started day after admission, when patient's condition has stabilized

Occupational Therapy

Second day admit activities are performed in bed, elbows supported, using only forearms and hands. Lasts 5 days or more depending on patient's progress

As the patient progresses in functional nursing activities he or she may work sitting in a straight-back chair in his room while doing occupational therapy activity (twice daily, work up to maximum of 20-min sessions).

Tile projects
Leather tooling
Linked belts
Stenciling
 Oil painting
Knitting
Crocheting
Model kit assembly
Cards, games, etc.
Embroidery

Nursing Activities

Turn in bed
Self-feeding
Brush teeth
Finish bath
Use commode
Shave
Chair b.i.d.

Recreation

Reading
Writing
Use telephone
Television
Radio

Physical Therapy

From day 2 of admission (following stabilization in CCU) through day 5, exercises are performed supine in bed.

AM: Active-assistive range-of-motion exercises × 5 to shoulders, elbows, wrists, hands

Diaphragmatic breathing exercises × 5

PM: Active-assistive range-of-motion exercises × 5 to hips, knees, ankles, toes
Active ankle circling, toe curling × 5 each

II. **Subacute Stage** (energy expenditure of 1.5–2.7 × basal metabolism): Started on the sixth day after admission

Nursing Activities

Sit in chair for gradually increasing periods of time
Brush teeth
Groom hair
Sponge bath
Walking in room

Occupational Therapy

By wheelchair to Cardiac Rehabilitation Room, located on the cardiac unit. Toward end of stage may walk to Cardiac Rehabilitation Room. Work in a group up to maximum of 30 min twice daily on bilateral light arm activities. Rx starting at 2:30 p.m. Examples:

Turkish rug knotting
Weaving on small loom
Rubber link mats
Leather carving, stamping, and lacing
Light sanding
Copper tooling

Needlework
Cord knotting
Block printing

Physical Therapy

Graded calisthenics (see procedure for calisthenics)
Exercises performed at 1.5–2.7 × basal metabolism

Sitting or standing depending on activity level of patient
Progress from 1 to 8 min b.i.d. as tolerated by patient
Metronome used to set correct speed and counts per minute
AM: Active range of motion to upper extremities × 5
PM: Active range of motion to lower extremities × 5

Ambulation in room as tolerated

III. *Convalescent Stage* (energy expenditure of 2.5–6.0 × basal metabolism):
Started on the 11th day.

Nursing Activities

Dressing
Bathroom privileges
Ambulation as ordered by physician
As patient progresses he or she is allowed to take showers

Occupational Therapy

Walk to Cardiac Rehabilitation room for 45 min session b.i.d. to start at
     2:00 p.m.
Bilateral arm activities with moderate resistance. Examples:
     Sawing ¼- or ½-inch wood with coping saw
     Metal hammering
Later: Bilateral arm activity with heavy resistance. Examples:
     Heavy woodworking (saw 1-inch wood with handsaw)
     Work with clay by hand
     Loom with 12 lb resistance

Physical Therapy

Graded calisthenics (see procedure for calisthenics)
     Exercises performed at 2.6–5.9 × basal metabolism
     Progress from 8 to 16 min b.i.d., as tolerated
     Perform standing
Ambulation progression from 50 feet to 200 feet.
Stair climbing on steps provided, progress from 3 to 12 steps
Optional—as ordered by physician
     Stationary bicycle without resistance, 5–20 min maximum
     Treadmill activity

IV. *Monitoring*

Electrocardiographic monitoring is performed at the completion of
each stage to determine if the patient is ready to progress to the next level of
activity.

IV. Monitoring test (monitoring takes the place of the patient's regular Occupational Therapy period)

Patient works in his or her room on an appropriate Occupational Therapy activity.

Readings are taken under nursing surveillance.

Physician reviews the EKG to determine if the patient may begin the next level of activity.

If the patient is not able to complete monitoring (see below) he or she remains at that level until the physician feels that the patient can retake the test.

1. End of the Acute Stage
   Patient is monitored at 1.3 × basal
   Tile project or Link belt for 20 min period
   EKG readings are taken before the patient begins and after every 4 min of work. Patient rests while the readings are taken.

2. End of the Subacute Stage
   Patient is monitored at 2.1 × basal
   Bilateral sanding with 4 lb resistance at a rate of 100 strokes/min
   Patient sands for 6 min—readings are taken after every 2 min of activity, patient rests for 4 min and readings are taken.

3. End of the Convalescent Stage
   Patient monitored at 2.9 × basal
   Patient must lift a weight from chair to a table to another chair at a rate of 46 moves/min:
   10 lb for men
   7 or 10 lb for women
   3 to 5 lb for some elderly patients
   Readings are taken in the same manner as for the subacute monitoring test.

Discontinue testing before test is completed if
ST depression 2 mm greater than at resting stage
Rate increase above 120 bpm
Increased number of PVCs (or other major arrhythmia)

Or if pain, shortage of breath, fatigue, etc.
Before each strip is run push the standardize button to "throw in" the 10 mm deflector to show that machine is standardized.

Tests are discontinued if patient complains or shows signs of excessive
Fatigue
Pain
Inability to continue
Perspiration, pale, moist facies
Heavy breathing

IV.   Shortness of breath, dyspnea on exertion
       Lightheadedness
       Tachycardia, palpitation
    If ECG changes are noted such as those listed below the test is stopped:
       Premature ventricular contractions
       Arrhythmias
       Signs of ischemia
       Abnormal increase in patient's pulse rate

V. *Discharge Instructions*

Individual home programs consisting of activities at different energy levels for various functional and recreational activities and calisthenics are given to patients with individual instruction. Also, vocational evaluations and counseling and psychosocial evaluations are conducted as prescribed prior to discharge and on an outpatient basis.

VI. *Weekends*

Patients may work in their rooms on projects below their present level of activity (e.g., if a patient progresses to convalescent activity before he or she finishes subacute level projects, they may be finished in the room at the patient's leisure). Work periods are limited to 20 minutes b.i.d. Patient may ambulate according to present activity level. A physical therapist will supervise exercise sessions on weekends.

A-2   Patient Information: Welcome to the Cardiac Rehabilitation Program

WELCOME

Your doctor has started you on the Cardiac Rehabilitation Program. The purpose of the program is to gradually increase your physical activity to assist you in returning to your normal activity level. In addition, you will be supplied with information about your heart attack, the healing process and how your future lifestyle may be affected. We are here to serve your needs. The following pages briefly describe the functions performed by various members of the cardiac rehabilitation team. We hope we can make your rehabilitation as safe and educational as possible. Feel free to contact any team member to assist you with questions or concerns you or your family may have.

Your activity level will be progressed through three stages—I, II, and III. Stage I begins with low level activities in bed, in Stage II your activities will be done sitting, and Stage III is done sitting, standing, and walking. You will be seen twice a day for specific activity sessions with Physical and Occupational Therapy: 10:30–12:00 a.m. and 2:15–4:30 p.m. The amount of time spent varies with your particular stage. Stages II and III require more time; therefore, they do begin before your rest period ends at 3:00.

In addition to these activity sessions, your doctor will gradually increase your daily activities from bedrest, up in a chair, and so on each day. If you are unsure of your activity limitations please ask. Your doctor also determines which therapy stage you begin on, and he will order your advancement to the next stage. You will be monitored with an EKG machine while performing a specific activity before you advance to a higher level.

Your exercise therapy will be closely supervised. Your pulse is taken before and after each activity. It is important for you to learn to take your own pulse. When you go home, *you* will be supervising your own activity. Caution must be taken not to overload the healing process of the heart. You should be sure to tell the therapist before, after, or during anytime you notice symptoms such as:

1. Chest pain
2. Severe headache, dizziness, and fainting
3. Irregular heart rate or palpitations
4. Extreme fatigue (exhaustion)
5. Nausea, vomiting, or diarrhea
6. Shortness of breath
7. Profuse sweating

These symptoms may indicate that your activities are too strenuous for your healing heart.

The program is based on a MET (metabolic equivalents) system. One MET is the amount of energy your body uses per minute at rest. All other activities are graded according to the energy required to perform that activity per minute.

Stage I = 1–1.5 METs   Stage II = 1.5–2.7 METs
Stage III = 2.6–4.0 METs

At the end of this handout you will find a listing of various activities and their estimated MET levels [see Tables 2.6–2.12].

A-3 Patient Information: The Physical Therapy Program

PHYSICAL THERAPY

Cardiac rehabilitation physical therapy consists of passive and active exercises that are supervised by a physical therapist. Initially, these exercises are performed while in bed primarily to aid blood circulation and to maintain muscle tone and flexibility. Gradual increased physical activities, including rhythmic calisthenic exercise, walking, and stair climbing, are performed during the remainder of the hospital stay.

Stage I exercises consist of active-assistive or active range-of-motion exercises to arms and legs, deep-breathing exercise, and active ankle motion while lying in bed.

Stage II exercises consist of calisthenics starting with 1 minute and increasing to 8 minutes while sitting in a chair, plus some active hip, knee, and ankle motions.

Stage III exercises consist of calisthenics beginning at 8 minutes and increasing to 16 minutes done while standing, and of supervised walking and stair climbing.

The Physical Therapy Home Program consists of the same calisthenic-type exercises that you perform while in the hospital with instruction for a gradual increase of activity and energy expenditure. There is also a structured walking program available if your physician wants you to participate in such a program.

Physical Therapy also offers an individualized outpatient rehabilitation program designed to improve your endurance and help you safely increase your physical activity to obtain a training effect. The program is run with 1–4 persons/session with constant monitoring by EKG leads, a physical therapist, and a registered nurse. Each session approximately 2 hours, 3 ×/week for 5 to 15 weeks. Your physician must order this service. If interested contact your physician, nurse, or therapist for details.

A-4 Patient Information: The Occupational Therapy Program

OCCUPATIONAL THERAPY

Occupational Therapy uses craft and recreational activities as a means of work substitution (instead of the normal activities you do at home or work). These activities have been evaluated so we know how much energy is expended as well as the specific type of exercise you get while performing the activity. The benefit of the activity is attributed only to the *exercise* derived from doing the activity. The workmanship of the particular project is irrelevant. The activity is determined according to the Stage you are on.

Stage I activities consist of light hand activities for a maximum of 20 minutes twice a day. This is done while you are sitting up in bed or in a chair in your room.

Stage II activities consist of activities involving both arms while sitting. You work for a maximum of 30 minutes twice a day. This is done in your room until you have bathroom privileges. Once you have bathroom privileges you can be brought to the Cardiac Rehabilitation Room on your floor via wheelchair to work on your activities.

Stage III activities consist of activities using both arms with resistance added. This stage involves both sitting and standing activities. You work for a maximum of 45 minutes twice a day. This activity is also done in the Cardiac Rehabilitation Room, where you will be taken via wheelchair until your doctor gives you appropriate walking privileges.

The Occupational Therapy Home Program is a guideline to show you how much of your normal daily activities you can be doing when you first go home from the hospital. It, too, is based on a gradual increase in your activity level.

A-5 *Patient Information: Educational Opportunities*

EDUCATIONAL OPPORTUNITIES

Cardiac Teacher

The cardiac teachers provide information to help you and your family live more comfortably and confidently with your heart problems. They will discuss with you the actual changes a heart goes through after a heart attack. They will discuss with you probable causes, treatment (including medications you may be taking), and future activity considerations during the healing process. All discussions and education sessions are open to family and friends you wish to include. There is a special support group for family members held on Thursdays form 2–3 p.m., where attendance is strongly suggested.

Educational Services Department has a selection of special educational programs available for private viewing. Programs must be ordered by your doctor. Contact your nurse if any of the following topics are of interest to you:

Coronary Angiography
Heart Attack: Recovery and Rehabilitation
Living With Angina Pectoris
Living With Heart Failure

Living With a Low Sodium Diet
Sex and the Heart Patient
Smoking: What Your Doctor Wants You to Know
High Blood Pressure: Introduction
How to Measure Blood Pressure
You Can Stop Smoking: Ways to Do It
Obesity
Relaxation Skills
Stress and Relaxation
Heart Risk Factors: Staying Well

Nutrition

A member of the nutrition staff will visit you during your hospital stay to discuss any modification of the diet prescribed by your doctor. Individual home diet instructions can be arranged with an order from your doctor. In addition, a weekly class of adding "spirit and spice to a modified diet" (low sodium, low cholesterol, low saturated fat, or calorie controlled) is given by a registered dietician for patients, their families, and friends. The class is held each Wednesday at 2:00 p.m. Ask your nurse for the location.

Social Service

The Social Service and Pastoral Care Departments are available to assist you and your family in social and emotional areas that are affected by your heart attack. The social worker, chaplain, and cardiac teacher co-support a group for family members of heart attack patients. Families are invited to share their concerns and gain an understanding of the heart attack and its effects. The group meets from 2:00 to 3:00 each Thursday. Ask your nurse for the location.

A-6   *The Physical Therapy Inpatient Cardiac Rehabilitation Program*

PHYSICAL THERAPY

Goal

To provide an individualized cardiovascular exercise program of graded movements evolving into a low intensity aerobics program which will develop cardiovascular conditioning and exercise tolerance to a level sufficient for return to the patient's home environment

To promote patient awareness for the body's need for and response to physical conditioning which will facilitate the incorporation of regular aerobic exercise into the patient's lifestyle

To supply basic information regarding the relationship of physical exertion and the healing myocardium to facilitate good judgment regarding independent activity selection at home

Rationale

Early mobilization minimizes the debilitating effects of bedrest—muscle atrophy, tachycardia with orthostatic hypotension, hypovolemia, thromboembolism, and decreased pulmonary ventilation.

Physical exercise, rhythmic calisthenics, and aerobics promote increased endurance and work capacity with a resultant increase in cardiovascular efficiency. Research has documented the physiologic parameters responsible such as decreased VO_2 for a given workload, decreased resting heart rates, improved peripheral circulation, etc.

Exercise can promote greater self-confidence, decrease anxiety, and enhance the patient's outlook toward a higher quality of life.

In total, the above factors promote a comprehensive recovery pattern resulting in decreased hospital stay.

Objectives

Mobilization initiated at CCU level
b.i.d. graded rhythmic calisthenics → ambulation → stairs
Optional bicycle or treadmill progression
Monitoring patient cardiovascular response
Documenting heart rate response
Optional home progams:
1. Progressive rhythmic calisthenics
2. Walking programs; liberal or conservative
3. Outpatient cardiac reconditioning program
Comprehensive introduction to program describing team approach
Supply handout of program components to patient and family
Instruction in radial pulse self-monitoring
Inform patient of pulse response each session
Discuss physiologic basis for patient's cardiovascular response
Explain MET sytem
Relate MET levels to activities of daily living (ADLs) and program stages
Supply listing of MET rated activities
Informal individual and/or group discussions:
1. Healing myocardium need for balanced rest and activity
2. Classical and individual cardiovascular warning symptoms
3. Isotonic (aerobic) versus isometric physiologic responses
4. Physiologic response to weather plus exercise
5. Benefits of cardiovascular training

Patients exercise in groups
Facilitate group interaction
Encourage family observation

PHYSICAL THERAPY CARDIAC PROGRAM

Stage I—CCU

Day 1-3   (day 2 after admission, patient stabilized)
   a.m.:   Active-assistive range of motion 5 × to upper extremities—shoulders, elbows, wrists, fingers, thumbs
   Breathing exercises, diaphragmatic, 5 ×

   p.m.:   Active-assistive range of motion 5 × to hips, knees, ankles, toes
   Active ankle circling and toe curling 5 × each

Days 4-5   Progress as tolerated to active range of motion starting with 5 ×, increasing two increments to a maximum 10 ×
   a.m.:   Active range of motion exercises 5 × each to shoulders, elbows, wrists, fingers, thumb
   Breathing exercises, diaphragmatic, 5 ×.

   p.m.:   Active range of motion exercises 5 × each to hips, knees, ankles, toes
   Active ankle circling and toe curling 5 × each

Stage II—Subacute

Exercises performed at 0.5–2.7 × basal metabolism
Perform sitting (once session 8 complete, may perform standing)
Progress from 1 to 8 min b.i.d. as tolerated
Metronome used to set correct speed and counts per minute

Day 6   Begin graded exercise program with rests PRN.
   Session 1 (a.m.)
   1 min exercise at 1.5 basal
   Rest as needed
   Total: 1 min exercise
   Active range of motion to lower extremities—hip flexion, knee extension, ankle circling 5 × each

   Session 2 (p.m.)
   1 min exercise at 1.5 basal
   Rest as needed
   1 min exercise at 2.1 basal
   Rest as needed
   Total: 2 min exercise
   Active range of motion to lower extremities—hip flexion, knee extension, ankle circling 5 × each

Day 7

   Session 3 (a.m.)

     1 min exercise each

     Rest as needed

     Use this time sequence at 1.5, 2.0, and 2.1 basal

     Total: 3 min exercise

     Active range of motion to lower extremities—hip flexion, knee extension, ankle circling 5 × each

Session 4 (p.m.)

     1 min exercise each

     Rest as needed

     Use this time sequence at 1.5, 1.9, 2.0, and 2.1 basal

     Total: 4 min exercise

     Active range of motion to lower extremities—hip flexion, knee extension, ankle circling 5 × each

Day 8

   Session 5 (a.m.)

     2 min exercise

     Rest as needed

     Use this time sequence at 2.0, 2.1, and 2.2 basal

     Total: 6 min exercise

     Active range of motion to lower extremities—hip flexion, knee extension, ankle circling 5 × each

   Session 6 (p.m.)

     Same as Session 5

     Active range of motion to lower extremities—hip flexion, knee extension, ankle circling 5 × each

Day 9

   Session 7 (a.m.)

     2 min exercise

     Minimal rest

     Use this time sequence at 2.0, 2.1, 2.3, and 2.7 basal

     Total: 8 min exercise

     Active range of motion to lower extremities—hip flexion, knee extension, ankle circling 5 × each

   Session 8 (p.m.)

     Use same time sequence as Session 7

     Use 2.0, 2.2, 2.3, and 2.7 basal

     Total: 8 min exercise

     Active range of motion to lower extremities—hip flexion, knee extension, ankle circling 5 × each

Stage III—Convalescent

     Exercises performed at 2.1–5.9 × basal metabolism

     Standing preferred

     Progress from 8 to 16 min b.i.d. as tolerated

Day 10
   2 min exercise
   Minimal rest
   Use this time sequence at 2.0, 2.1, 2.3, 2.7, and 2.8 basal
   Total: 10 min exercise
   Ambulation: 50 feet

Day 11
   Use same time sequence as day 10 at 2.1, 2.3, 2.6, 2.8, and 3.2 basal
   Total: 10 min exercise
   Ambulation: 50 feet

Day 12
   Exercise at 2.1, 2.2, 2.3, 2.6, 2.8, and 3.2 basal
   Total: 12 min exercise
   Ambulation: 100 feet
   Progress to stairs: 3 steps

Day 13
   Exercise at 2.2, 2.3, 2.6, 2.7, 2.8, and 3.2 basal
   Total: 12 min exercise
   Ambulation: 100 feet
   Stairs: 3 steps

Day 14
   Exercise at 2.2, 2.3, 2.6, 2.7, 2.8, 3.2, and 3.6 basal
   Total: 14 min exercise
   Ambulation: 150 feet
   Stairs: 3 steps

Day 15
   Exercise at 2.2, 2.6, 2.8, 3.2, 3.6, and 5.0 basal
   Total: 14 min exercise
   Ambulation: 150 feet
   Stairs: 3 steps

Day 16
   Exercise at 2.2, 2.6, 2.7, 2.8, 3.2, 3.6, 5.0, and 5.9 basal
   Total: 16 min exercise
   Ambulation: 200 feet
   Stairs: 6 steps

Day 17
   Same as day 16, until discharge

Notes

   Bicycle and treadmill optional
   Patient is held at any specific exercise level or exercise is reduced if patient fatigues or if adverse symptoms are noted (see precaution sheet).

A-7 Rehabilitation Calisthenics for Stage II and Stage III of the Cardiac Rehabilitation Program

STAGE II Sitting

No#	Each Position Equals One Count					Count Min	METS	Hints
	1	2	3	4	5			
1						66	1.5	Bend at the waist
2						90	2.1	Stretch arms out at 3
3						112	1.9	Very fast forward and back equal one count
4						66	2.0	Side stretch at 2, 4
5						80	2.7	Twist your trunk Stretch arms
6						66	2.3	Keep elbows straight
7						112	2.3	Fast. Elbows straight 2, 4

STAGE III Standing

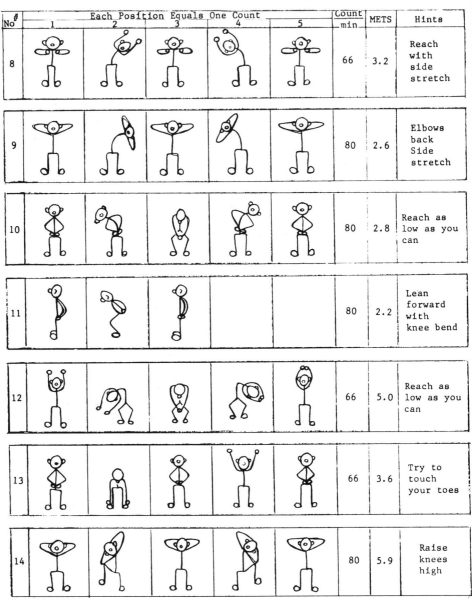

No#	Each Position Equals One Count					Count min	METS	Hints
	1	2	3	4	5			
8						66	3.2	Reach with side stretch
9						80	2.6	Elbows back Side stretch
10						80	2.8	Reach as low as you can
11						80	2.2	Lean forward with knee bend
12						66	5.0	Reach as low as you can
13						66	3.6	Try to touch your toes
14						80	5.9	Raise knees high

MET values for calisthenics 1–11 and 13 were determined by interpolation from experimentally determined heart rate and MET relationship.

MET values for calisthenics 12 and 14 were taken from Amundsen L, et al.: Energy cost of rehabilitation calisthenics. Phy Ther 59:855, 1979.

A-8   Form for Recording Pulse Rate

PHYSICAL THERAPY
CARDIAC REHABILITATION

THERAPIST _____
CODE _____

PULSE RECORD BEFORE/AFTER EXERCISE

Stage I (Days 1-5)   Supine   Active-assistance ROM—Active ROM   Breathing   Foot Exercises

| Date/therapist code |
| AAROM U.E. Breathing |
| AAROM L.E. Foot Exercises |
| AROM U.E. Breathing |
| AROM L.E. Foot Exercises |

Stage II (Days 6-9)   Sitting   Arm Exercise   1–8 min   1.2–2.6 METs   Active ROM   Lower Extremities

| Date/Therapist Code |
| 1 min   1.5 METs |
| 2 min   1.5–1.9 METs |
| 3 min   1.5–2.0 METs |
| 4 min   1.5–2.0 METs |
| 6 min   2.0–2.3 METs |
| 6 min   2.0–2.3 METs |
| 8 min   2.0–2.3 METs |
| 8 min   2.0–2.7 METs |

Stage III (Days 10–16)   Standing   Arm, Trunk Exercise   2.1–4.1 METs   50–100 feet Ambulation   Steps

| Date/Therapist Code |
| 10 min   2.0–2.8 METs, 50 ft |
| 10 min   2.1–3.2 METs, 50 ft |
| 12 min   2.1–3.2 METs, 100 ft, 3 steps |
| 12 min   2.2–3.2 METs, 100 ft, 3 steps |
| 14 min   2.2–3.6 METs, 150 ft, 3 steps |
| 14 min   2.2–5.0 METs, 200 ft, 6 steps |
| 16 min   2.2–5.9 METs, 200 ft, 6 steps |

A circled box indicates an abnormal exercise response. Explanation in progress notes on back of this form.

Name _____ **Hospital No.** _____

[*The section below is printed on the back of the form*]

Physician _____ **Diagnosis** _____
Date of Onset _____ **Self-Monitoring Pulse (Yes/No)** _____
Initial Note and Progress Notes:

[*ROM, range of motion; AAROM, active-assistive ROM; AROM, active ROM; U.E., upper extremity; L.E., lower extremity*]

HURRAH ... YOU'RE GOING HOME!

These exercises are an ongoing progression from your hospital exercise program. It is important to gradually increase your activity during the first few weeks at home as you begin to resume your normal activities. Be conscientious with your exercises. You and your heart deserve the best!

GENERAL GUIDELINES

1. Exercise twice each day.
2. Do not exercise directly after meals; wait 1½ to 2 hours. Better yet, exercise just before a meal.
3. Start the exercises the day *after* you get home.
4. Begin with the set marked by your therapist.
5. Each set (a–n) contains a series of exercises (1–14) They are illustrated by number on the attached sheets.
6. Note each exercise's individual cadence number. The speed is important to control the energy you put out.
7. Do each set for 3–4 days. Advance to the next set unless you have experienced excessive fatigue, shortness of breath, or chest discomfort.
8. Call your doctor if you experience chest pain.
9. If you are ill and/or miss some exercise sessions, start again at the next lower set.
10. Keep advancing every 3–4 days. Report your progress at your doctor's appointments. Together you can plan future activity.

EXERCISE SPECIFICS

Stage II
All exercises are done *sitting*
Exercises a–d are 1 minute each
Exercises e–n are 2 minutes each

Set	Exercises	Total Minutes
a.	1	1
b.	1,2	2
c.	1,2,3	3
d.	1,2,3,4,	4
e.	3,4,5	6
f.	3,4,5,6,	8
g.	4,5,6,7,	8

Stage III
All exercises are done *standing*
All exercises are 2 minutes each

Set	Exercises	Total Minutes
h.	4,5,6,7,8	10
i.	5,6,7,8,9	10
j.	5,6,7,8,9,10	12
k.	6,7,8,9,10,11	12
l.	6,7,8,9,10,11,12	14
m.	7,8,9,10,11,12,13	14
n.	7,8,9,10,11,12,13,14	16

Additional Comments:

Name _____   Any questions?
Therapist _____   Call 932-5486
Date _____   Physical Therapy
                                      Methodist Hospital

A-10 *Patient Information: Walking Schedules*

GENERAL GUIDELINES

1. Walking should be done on the level.
2. Walking should be done once daily to increase your fitness level.
3. Do not walk immediately after meals, and use good sense in regard to weather conditions, temperature, and humidity.
4. Do not walk if you are having any of the following symptoms:
    Excessive fatigue
    Chest pain
    Lightheadedness or dizziness, severe headache
    Irregular heart rate or palpitations
    Nausea or vomiting
    Shortness of breath
5. Take a 10 second pulse at end of walk—it should not exceed 115 beats/min. If it does or if you have adverse symptoms, contact your physician.
6. 1 block = 1 long block = 650 feet = ⅛ mile

WALKING SCHEDULE A

Week	Round-Trip Distance (Blocks)	(Miles)	One-Way Distance (Blocks)	Approx. Speed and Time (min.)
1	(around house and yard as desired)			(slowly—2 mph)
2	1	⅛	½	3¾
3	2	¼	1	7½
4	4	½	2	15
5	6	¾	3	22½
6	8	1	4	30
7	8	1	4	(moderately—3 mph)
8	8	1	4	20
9	10	1¼	5	25
10	12	1½	6	30
11	12	1½	6	(briskly—4 mph)
12	12	1½	6	22½
13	14	1¾	7	26
14	14	1¾	7	26
15	16	2	8	30
16	16	2	8	30

WALKING SCHEDULE B

Week	Round-Trip Distance (Blocks)	(Miles)	One-Way Distance (Blocks)	Approx. Speed and Time (min.)
1	(around house and yard as desired)			(slowly—2 mph)
2	2	¼	1	7½
3	4	½	2	15
4	8	1	4	30
5	12	1½	6	45
6	16	2	8	60
7	16	2	8	(moderately—3 mph)
8	16	2	8	40
9	20	2½	10	50
10	24	3	12	60
11	24	3	12	(briskly—4 mph)
12	24	3	12	45
13	28	3½	14	52
14	28	3½	14	52
15	32	4	16	60
16	32	4	16	60

Appendix B

*Outpatient Cardiac Rehabilitation
Program
Department of Rehabilitation Medicine
Physical Therapy
Methodist Hospital
St. Louis Park, Minn.*

TABLE OF CONTENTS

B-1   An Overview of the Outpatient Cardiac Rehabilitation Program (OCRP)

GOAL

To provide an outpatient cardiac rehabilitation program for a selected group of cardiac patients for optimal rehabilitation of the individual to her or his fullest physical potential

This will be attained by development of cardiovascular conditioning, improvement of physical fitness and exercise tolerance, increasing patient knowledge of the disease process, and development of positive psychological adjustment. Individual exercise levels will be set from the results of the exercise EKG test which will be performed prior to initiation of the program.

PROGRAM CONTENT

Exercise Testing Guidelines

Naughton's Protocol   Recommended for patients who may not tolerate a full Bruce test and for those with recent MIs, using heart rate limits based on the period of time post MI:

2 weeks—120 bpm
3 weeks—130 bpm
5 weeks—140 bpm
7 weeks—150 bpm

Bruce's Protocol   A maximal symptom limited test is recommended for patients 9 weeks or more post MI and for most patient referrels with other diagnoses.

Exercise Training

Training Workload Levels   Under ideal conditions 75 percent of the MET level achieved on maximal symptom limited treadmill test is needed to gain any objective improvement in exercise tolerance. In patients with angina, arrhythmias, or other problems this may need modification. As the patient's tolerance to exercise improves, the training workload should be slowly increased.

Maximum training heart rate will be 85 percent of maximum treadmill heart rate following a symptom limited stress test.

Type of Activity   Ergometers (biking); treadmill (walking).

Frequency   Patients will be seen approximately 1½ hours 3 times a week

Duration   5, 10, or 15 weeks. It is recommended that a patient achieve and tolerate training at an 8 MET level before being discharged from the program.

Education

Anatomy and Physiology of the Heart   Chambers, coronary arteries, disease process, collateral circulation, angina

Risk Factors   Hypertension, smoking, diet, overweight, anxiety/stress, sedentary lifestyle

Medications

Physiology of Exercise

Effects and Components of Cardiovascular Training

Cardiac Adjustment Group [Optional]

To establish a supportive reference group in which the cardiac patient can learn and test new behaviors and deal with the emotional impact of the disease upon the individual, the family, employment, and lifestyle. The group will be conducted by a Registered Clinical Social Worker and will meet once a week.

Dietary Consultation [Optional]

A dietician is available for diet instruction or specific diet problems.

PROGRAM PROCEDURES

Monitoring

Progress will be evaluated by supine and sitting pulse and blood pressure at the beginning of each exercise session and at 5 min intervals thereafter. At every exercise session a graph flow sheet on each patient will be kept. EKG monitor strips will be taken before and after exercise and at appropriate intervals during exercise.

Exercise Sessions

Week 1

Introduce patient to program procedures and staff, exercise warning signs, education, and available services

Exercise will begin according to protocol and prescription:

Calisthenics warm-ups

Exercise at 1.5–3.6 METs for 4 min

Warm-up on bike ergometer or treadmill

Warm-ups will be done at one-third of training workload for 2 min followed by 1 min rest

Increase to two-thirds of training workload for 2 min followed by 1 min rest

Training

With workload based on exercise prescription, training will consist of six repetitions of 2 min work followed by 1 min rest

Cool-down on bike ergometer or treadmill

Exercise performed at two-thirds of training workload for 2 min followed by 1 min rest and then one-third of workload for 2 min followed by 1 min rest

Calisthenic Cool-down

Exercise from 1.5 to 3.6 METs for 4 min

Week 2 Through Discharge

Exercise Sessions   There will be a weekly increase of training MET level or repetitions in the training period, and heart rate limits will be raised according to patient tolerance, OCRP guidelines, and physician prescription

Progress Reports   Reports will be sent to the patient's physician upon completion of each 5 weeks

Home Programs   Upon discharge, a home program using heart rate and workload guidelines from patient's record at OCRP is available to patient and physician

Followup   A followup questionnaire will be sent to each patient 2 weeks after discharge from OCRP. This will be followed by a phone call in 2–4 weeks. In addition, followup on a monthly basis is available for a patient to come to OCRP to exercise while monitored on EKG, to discuss problems or questions, and to update the home program.

EXERCISE PRECAUTIONS:

Abnormal Responses to Increased Intensity of Work

Blood Pressure

Failure to rise (systolic pressure)

Progressive fall in systolic pressure

Heart Rate

Excessive tachycardia

Bradycardia

EKG

Ischemic deviation of ST segments (depression or elevation)

Arrhythmias, ventricular tachycardia, multifocal ventricular premature contractions, atrial tachyarrhythmia, atrioventricular block greater than first degree

Symptoms

Anginal pain

Inappropriate breathlessness

Faintness, dizziness, lightheadedness, confusion

Leg pain (claudication)

Signs
  Cyanosis, pallor, mottling of skin
  Cold sweat, piloerection
  Ataxia, glassy stare
  Gallop heart sounds
  Valvular regurgitative murmur
  Abnormal cardiac impulse
Other Precautions
  Inderal use
  Pacemaker—if cannot increase heart rate
  Drugs to decrease heart rate

Symptoms and Signs of Exercise Effort—Indications for Reduction of Exercise Intensity

During Exercise and Immediately Thereafter
  Anginal discomfort
  Ataxia, lightheadedness, confusion
  Nausea, vomiting
  Leg claudication
  Pallor, cyanosis
  Dyspnea persisting for more than 10 min
  Arrhythmias
  Inappropriate bradycardia
Delayed
  Prolonged fatigue
  Insomnia
  Weight gain due to fluid retention–heart failure
  Persistent tachycardia (heart rate should be below 120 bpm at 6 min after exercise; higher intensities and durations of effort have longer recovery times)

DISCONTINUATIONS:

Reasons for Temporarily Reducing or Deferring Exercise Training

  Intercurrent illness—febrile, injury, GI
  Progression of cardiac disease
  Orthopedic problem
  Emotional turmoil
  Severe sunburn
  Alcoholic hangover
  Cerebral dysfunction—dizziness, vertigo
  Sodium retention—edema, weight gain

Dehydration

Environmental factors—weather (excessive heat or cold, humidity, or wind); air pollution (smog, CO)

Overindulgence—large, heavy meal within 2 hours; coffee, tea, cola (xanthines and other stimulating beverages)

Drugs—decongestants, bronchodilators, atropine, weight reducers (anorectics)

Indications for Discontinuing Exercise Training Program

Orthopedic problems, aggravated by activity
Progression of cardiac illness unresponsive to medical therapy
Development of new systemic disease aggravated by exercise
Major surgery
Psychiatric decompensation
Acute alcoholism

PATIENT SELECTION

Coronary Heart Disease
  Angina pectoris
  Myocardial infarction
  Postoperative vein bypass
  Postventricular aneurysm resection
Nonischemic Heart Disease
  Postoperative valvular patients
  Mild mitral stenosis—cardiac rehabilitation is not indicated in aortic insufficiency and is contraindicated in aortic stenosis
  Congenital heart disease—atrial septal defect with normal pulmonary vascular resistance; ventricular septal defect without pulmonary hypertension
  Hypertensive cardiovascular disease
  Peripheral vascular disease
Potential Heart Disease
  Presence of coronary risk factors
  Sinus tachycardia and hyperkinetic states
  Chronic lung disease, obstructive rather than restrictive
Subclinical Heart Disease
  EKG ischemic manifestations—individuals without symptoms upon exercise testing
  Abnormal resting EKG—interpreted as showing a healed silent MI or injury of unspecified type

CONTRAINDICATIONS TO EXERCISE TRAINING AND EXERCISE TESTING

Acute Illness Includes respiratory, GI, or other febrile illness; phlebitis and embolism

Active, Chronic, Systemic Disease (Uncontrolled) Includes thyroid, renal, hepatic, rheumatic disease, gout, etc.

Anatomic Abnormalities Uncompensated valvular heart disease; gross cardiomegaly

Functional Abnormalities Arrhythmias; ventricular tachycardia; uncontrolled atrial fibrillation; second and third degree heart block

STAFFING

M.D. A cardiologist or the referring physician will be responsible for directing and interpreting the stress test. Referral and prescriptions must be written by a physician. The Medical Advisor for the OCRP will be available for consultation on all patients.

OCRP Staff A minimum of two staff people will be present at all times, *a physical therapist and an R.N., both trained in CPR and emergency procedures. They will be responsible for supervising the exercise session* and monitoring the EKG and vital signs throughout. No more than four patients will be treated at a given time.

LOCATION

The program is located in the Outpatient Cardiac Rehabilitation Room in the Physical Therapy Department.

B-2 Outpatient Cardiac Rehabilitation Referral Form

I. Name _____ Age _____ Sex _____
Address _____ Zip _____
Occupation _____ Phone: # Home _____ Work _____

II. *The Full Outpatient Cardiac Rehabilitation Program Includes:*
EKG stress test on treadmill prior to beginning training
Calisthenics; warmup, training, and cooldown on bicycle each session
Monitored blood pressure, heart rate, EKG strips during training

Patient education classes, retests, and home programs
Optional adjustment group
Dietary consultation available
Monthly followup

III. *Goal:* Develop cardiovascular conditioning, improve physical fitness and exercise tolerance, and increase patient's knowledge of disease process

IV. *Indications for Cardiac Rehabilitation*
_____ Myocardial Infarction
      Date and Site of First MI _____
      Second MI _____
      Third MI _____
      Complications of MI
         _____ Shock
         _____ CHF
         _____ Anneurysm foundation
         _____ Pericarditis
         _____ Arrhythmias
         Type and frequency _____
_____ Angina
      Approx. date of onset _____
      Relief with nitroglycerin _____
      Frequency _____
      Recent changes indicating unstable
      pattern _____
_____ Cardiac surgery—Date and type _____

V. *Other Relevant Diagnoses*

VI. *Current Medications and Dosage*
1. _____ 3. _____
2. _____ 4. _____
Serum potassium value with date if on a diuretic: _____

VII. *Current Diet* _____

VIII. *Risk Factors*
_____ Hypertension
_____ Smoking—Duration _____ Amount _____
_____ Cholesterol level _____
_____ Triglyceride level _____
_____ Diabetes

IX. *Special Precautions and Recommendations:*

X. *Prescription*
Duration of program: _____ 5 weeks _____ 10 weeks _____ 15 weeks
Training MET level you desire for patient_____
Under ideal conditions 75 percent of the MET level achieved on maximal symptom limited treadmill test is needed to gain any objective improvement in exercise tolerance. In patients with angina, arrhythmias, or other special problems, this may need modification. Maximum training heart rate will be 85 percent of maximum treadmill heart rate following a symptom limited stress test. Please attach copy of treadmill test.
_____ Patient may participate in optional adjustment group if desired
_____ Please arrange for dietary consult
_____ Please refer to Dr. _____ for exercise prescription
[may be filled out by cardiologist monitoring treadmill test]

Primary Physician _____ **Date** _____
Office Phone Number _____

B-3 *Informed Consent for Exercise Treatment*

I desire to engage voluntarily in the outpatient cardiac exercise program in order to improve my cardiovascular function as recommended to me by my physician Dr. _____.

Before I enter this exercise program I will have a clinical evaluation consisting of but not limited to measurements of heart rate and blood pressure, electrocardiogram at rest and with effort. The purpose of this evaluation is to detect any condition which would indicate that I should not engage in this exercise program.

The program will follow an exercise prescription prepared by Dr. _____ and will be carefully followed by the supervisor of the exercise program and regulated to my tolerance. The activities are designed to place a gradually increasing workload on the circulation and thereby improve its function. There is the risk of unpredictable changes occurring during or following the exercise. These changes include abnormalities of blood pressure or heart rate, or ineffective "heart function" and in rare instances "heart attacks" or "cardiac arrest."

Before starting the program I will be instructed as to the signs and symptoms which I should report promptly to the supervisor of the exercises and which would alert me to modify my activities. Every effort will be made to avoid such events by the preliminary medical exam and by observation during the exercise. Emergency equipment and trained personnel are available to deal with unusual situations should they occur.

I have read the foregoing and I understand it. Any questions which may have occurred to me have been answered to my satisfaction.

Date _____

Patient Signature _____

Witness _____

B-4   *Patient Preinstruction Sheet: Outpatient Cardiac Rehabilitation Program*

Many studies have shown that individuals with heart disease can get the same beneficial effect from a conditioning program as normal individuals. However, it is much safer for cardiac patients to exercise under medical supervision.

Although there is no firm evidence that life will be prolonged or heart attacks prevented, we can assure that almost everyone who participates in this program will have more endurance and be capable of greater ability to work and enjoy life, with fewer symptoms.

There are several principles that you should understand prior to starting in an exercise program:

1. Exercise should be carried out three times weekly at an appropriate intensity and duration in order to achieve a "training effect." Exercise cannot be stored, and some of the gains will be lost if more than 2 days elapse between training sessions.

2. Attendance should be regular, although we realize that an occasional session will have to be missed because of illness, vacation, etc. If you are unable to attend, please call to notify staff at 932-6097.

3. People with infections such as bad colds or viral gastrointestinal upsets should not exercise.

4. If at any time during the exercise session you have chest discomfort or any unusual symptoms, you should notify the staff. Although many types of discomfort are experienced that are noncardiac, it is best to stop exercise until the discomfort can be evaluated.

5. You will find that as your conditioning improves, your cardiac or pulse rate may be lower.

Goals will be set for each individual and will be flexible, depending on progress. Progress will be slow and gradual. Each person will have an individual exercise prescription based on his or her latest exercise stress test. Stress tests will be repeated as indicated.

Many people believe they can initiate and carry out an exercise program on their own. This is rarely possible because self-discipline usually breaks down. The knowledge that a regular appointment must be kept to engage in exercise and that exercise will be carried out with a congenial group is usually the motivating factor that maintains exercise regularly.

We hope that exercise will become a permanent part of your life. Upon completion of the outpatient rehabilitation program, your physician will have the option of prescribing a diversified home program for you.

Various group education sessions will be offered to you in an effort to increase knowledge and acceptance of your condition. Such topics as exercise and activity levels, risk factors, diet, and psychological and social adjustments will be discussed by appropriate professionals.

INSTRUCTIONS FOR EXERCISE SESSIONS

1. Plan to be in the laboratory for 1 to 1½ hours.
2. Do not eat a heavy meal for at least 2 hours before exercise. The preceding meal should be light, without butter or cream, coffee, tea, or alcohol.
3. Continue taking your medications as usual.
4. Wear or bring appropriate clothing. Sneakers or walking shoes are needed (*no* slippers).

   Men: Should bring gym shorts, Bermuda shorts or a pair of loose-fitting, light trousers.

   Women: Should bring or wear a bra; short-sleeved, loose-fitting blouse that buttons in the front; and slacks, shorts, or even pajama pants. No one-piece undergarments or pantyhose are to be worn.

B-5 Outpatient Cardiac Rehabilitation Program Admitting Questionnaire

Please answer if applicable to you

1. Do you understand purpose and format of the Outpatient Cardiac Rehabilitation Program?

2. Are you presently on an exercise program?

   Of what type? What amount of time spent on it?

3. Do you know the coronary disease risk factors and which of these pertain to you?

4. What problems, if any, have you encountered at home (diet, exercise, etc.)?

5.   Would you like specific instructions or review of disease process, medical terms, exercise routines, or other related topics?

6.   Do you have any known allergies?

7.   Are you on a special diet?
     If so, what type?

     What problems, if any, have you encountered with it?

     Are you interested in further consultation with a dietician?

B-6 Outpatient Cardiac Exercise Training Program

				Exercise Time (min)							
Weeks	Intensity (kpm)	Ratio Work:Rest	Repetitions	Warm-up Calisthenics	Bike Warm-ups	Bike Training	Bike Cool-down	Cool-down Calisthenics	Total Exercise Time	Rest	Total Treatment Time
1		2:1	6	4	4	12	4	4	28	14	42
2		2:1	7	4	4	14	4	4	30	15	45
3		2:1	8	4	4	16	4	4	32	16	48
4		2:1	9	4	4	18	4	4	34	17	51
5		2:1	10	4	4	20	4	4	36	18	54
6		3:2	6	4	4	18	4	4	34	20	54
7		3:2	7	4	4	21	4	4	37	22	59
8		3:2	8	4	4	24	4	4	40	24	64
9		3:2	9	4	4	27	4	4	43	26	69
10		3:2	10	4	4	30	4	4	46	28	74
11		4:2	6	4	4	24	4	4	40	20	60
12		4:2	7	4	4	28	4	4	44	22	66
13		4:2	8	4	4	32	4	4	48	24	72
14		4:2	9	4	4	36	4	4	52	26	78
15		4:2	10	4	4	40	4	4	56	28	84

B-7 Outpatient Cardiac Rehabilitation Program Example: Maximum Work Capacity 600 kpm/min

Week		Calisthenics	Bike Warm-up	Bike Training	Bike Cool-down	Calisthenics
1	I	Recheck maximum on bike with M.D.				
	II	4 min	2 min at 150 kpm / 2 min at 300 kpm	12 min at 450 kpm at 2:1	2 min at 300 kpm / 2 min at 150 kpm	4 min
	III	4 min	2 min at 150 kpm / 2 min at 300 kpm	12 min at 450 kpm at 2:1	2 min at 300 kpm / 2 min at 150 kpm	4 min
2	I	4 min	2 min at 150 kpm / 2 min at 300 kpm	14 min at 450 kpm at 2:1	2 min at 300 kpm / 2 min at 150 kpm	4 min
	II	4 min	2 min at 150 kpm / 2 min at 300 kpm	14 min at 450 kpm at 2:1	2 min at 300 kpm / 2 min at 150 kpm	4 min
	III	4 min	2 min at 150 kpm / 2 min at 300 kpm	14 min at 450 kpm at 2:1	2 min at 300 kpm / 2 min at 150 kpm	4 min
3		Same at each session	Same at each session	16 min at 450 kpm at 2:1 at each session	Same at each session	Same at each session
4		Same	Same	18 min at 450 kpm at 2:1	Same	Same
5		Same	Same	20 min at 450 kpm at 2:1	Same	Same
6		Same	Same	18 min at 450 kpm at 3:2	Same	Same
7		Same	Same	21 min at 450 kpm at 3:2	Same	Same
8		4 min	2 min at 150 kpm / 2 min at 300 kpm	24 min at 450 kpm at 3:2	2 min at 300 kpm / 2 min at 150 kpm	4 min
9		Same	Same	27 min at 450 kpm at 3:2	Same	Same
10		Same	Same	30 min at 450 kpm at 3:2	Same	Same
11		Same	Same	24 min at 450 kpm at 4:2	Same	Same
12		Same	Same	28 min at 450 kpm at 4:2	Same	Same
13		Same	Same	32 min at 450 kpm at 4:2	Same	Same
14		Same	Same	36 min at 450 kpm at 4:2	Same	Same
15		Same	Same	40 min at 450 kpm at 4:2	Same	Same

B-8 Form for Graphing Pulse and Blood Pressure Responses

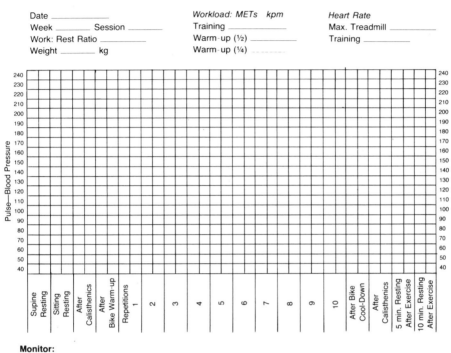

Date _____
Week _____ Session _____
Work: Rest Ratio _____
Weight _____ kg

Workload: METs kpm
Training _____
Warm-up (½) _____
Warm-up (¼) _____

Heart Rate
Max. Treadmill _____
Training _____

Monitor:

Comments:

Name _____

Hosp. No. _____

Hosp. R. No. _____

B-9   Outpatient Cardiac Rehabilitation Program Followup Statistics

Name:
Hosp. No.:
Date:
Phone or Visit?

Exercise
   Type
   Frequency
   Duration
   Work/rest
   Workload
Training Heart Rate
   Self-monitored
   Mechanical
Following Diet
   Low cholesterol
   Low sodium
   Low calorie
   Comments
Smoking—Quantity
Weight
Working—job
   Full or part time?
   Comments
Angina Frequency
   Comments
Medication Use
   1.   Nitroglycerin
   2.
   3.
   4.
Comments

Index